MDCT Physics

The Basics—Technology, Image Quality and Radiation Dose

Mahadevappa Mahesh, MS, PhD, FAAPM

Associate Professor and Chief Physicist
The Russell H. Morgan Department of Radiology and Radiological Science
Johns Hopkins University School of Medicine
Baltimore, MD

Wolters Kluwer | Lippincott Williams & Wilkins
Health

Philadelphia · Baltimore · New York · London
Buenos Aires · Hong Kong · Sydney · Tokyo

Acquisitions Editor: Brian Brown
Managing Editor: Ryan Shaw
Project Manager: Alicia Jackson
Senior Manufacturing Manager: Benjamin Rivera
Senior Marketing Manager: Angela Panetta
Designer: Stephen Druding
Cover Designer: TBA
Production Service: Cadmus Communications

Printed in China

Library of Congress Cataloging-in-Publication Data
ISBN: 9780781768115
ISBN: 078176811X
    Mahesh, Mahadevappa.
    MDCT Physics: The Basics—Technology, Image Quality and Radiation Dose / Mahadevappa Mahesh.
        p. ; cm.
    Includes bibliographical references.
    ISBN-13: 978-0-7817-6811-5
    ISBN-10: 0-7817-6811-X
    1. Tomography. 2. Medical physics. I. Title.
    [DNLM: 1. Tomography, X-Ray Computed. 2. Radiation Dosage. 3. Technology, Radiologic. 4. Tomography Scanners, X-Ray Computed. WN 206 M214c 2009]
    RC78.7.T6M34 2009
    616.07′57—dc22   2009006242

Care has been taken to confirm the accuracy of the information presented and to describe generally accepted practices. However, the authors, editors, and publisher are not responsible for errors or omissions or for any consequences from application of the information in this book and make no warranty, expressed or implied, with respect to the currency, completeness, or accuracy of the contents of the publication. Application of the information in a particular situation remains the professional responsibility of the practitioner.

The authors, editors, and publisher have exerted every effort to ensure that drug selection and dosage set forth in this text are in accordance with current recommendations and practice at the time of publication. However, in view of ongoing research, changes in government regulations, and the constant flow of information relating to drug therapy and drug reactions, the reader is urged to check the package insert for each drug for any change in indications and dosage and for added warnings and precautions. This is particularly important when the recommended agent is a new or infrequently employed drug.

Some drugs and medical devices presented in the publication have Food and Drug Administration (FDA) clearance for limited use in restricted research settings. It is the responsibility of the health care provider to ascertain the FDA status of each drug or device planned for use in their clinical practice.

To purchase additional copies of this book, call our customer service department at (800) 638-3030 or fax orders to (301) 223-2320. International customers should call (301) 223-2300.

Visit Lippincott Williams & Wilkins on the Internet: at LWW.com. Lippincott Williams & Wilkins customer service representatives are available from 8:30 am to 6 pm, EST.

10 9 8 7 6 5 4 3 2 1

*This book is dedicated to my beloved wife, Vasantha, and
to my lovely kids, Ajay and Smitha!*

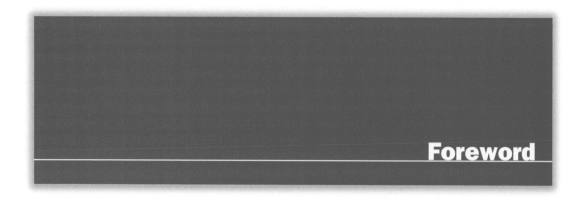

Elliot K. Fishman MD

The evolution of CT from single slice spiral CT through 4-slice MDCT, to 16-slice MDCT, to 64-slice MDCT, to dual source and beyond has changed the face of radiology and medicine in general by providing the unprecedented accuracy in lesion detection and characterization. Applications that were classic like evaluation of renal masses or pancreatic masses can be done more accurately, and new applications like virtual colonoscopy or cardiac CTA are the result of the new technology. Yet, these achievements are soon surpassed by even newer technologies ranging from 256- or 320-row detector scanners, to new high-resolution scanners, to the newest subsecond scanners that image in a flash. Not surprisingly, with these changes comes the demand for books on the key clinical topics, and a number of books have been published addressing these topics.

Although most of the larger clinical textbooks do provide a chapter or two on CT technology, these chapters are often diluted and cover only a minimum of facts or provide the information in a less than optimal format. For several years now, there has been the need for an up-to-date textbook on the physics of MDCT presented in a comprehensive yet easy-to-read format. Whether the reader is a radiologist, fellow, resident, or radiologic technologist, there is the need for information on topics ranging from principles of the different MDCT scanners, to improving image quality, to issues surrounding radiation dose.

To meet this need, Mahadevappa Mahesh has written a book that provides the answers to the most important topics in CT physics today. The title of the book says it all and more, *MDCT Physics: The Basics—Technology, Image Quality and radiation Dose*. The book covers not only the current issues in CT technology today, but also some future issues like dual energy CT and perfusion scanning. Hybrid systems, like PET-CT, are also clearly addressed.

The user will find this book easy to read but also comprehensive. Whether you are new in CT, or have years of experience and want to be brought up to speed on the state of the art, this book is for you. I congratulate Mahesh on a job well done.

Foreword

William Hendee, PhD

The introduction of x-ray computed tomography (CT) by Electro-Musical Instruments, Ltd. (EMI) in the early 1970s stimulated a rapid evolution in CT technology through four generations in just a few years. By the mid-1970s CT units employed a rotating x-ray tube and detector bank (3rd generation) or an x-ray tube rotating within a ring of stationary detectors (4th generation). Within a few years, a 5th generation geometry was introduced (electron-beam CT) in which a rotating electron beam generated a moving x-ray source, surrounding the patient. CT quickly replaced some other imaging technologies (e.g., pneumoencephalography and nuclear brain scans) and rapidly became a mainstay of medical imaging for medical diagnosis. CT was also found to be exceptionally useful in radiation therapy, and CT simulators for treatment planning were integrated expeditiously into radiation–oncology clinics of even modest size.

Over the 1980s and 1990s, CT experienced slow and steady growth as new clinical applications were found and additional technical features were developed. Then at the turn of the century, a major technical advance occurred, greatly facilitating the use of CT. This advance was the development of slip-ring technology so that the x-ray tube of 3rd generation CT units could rotate continuously in one direction around the patient as the patient was moved along the axis of the CT unit. This advance was termed "helical" or "spiral" CT scanning, and was soon joined by a second major technical advance, the use of multiple-detector arrays to produce several (up to 64 and more) CT slices simultaneously. The resulting multiple-row detector CT units (MDCT) have greatly enhanced the value of computed tomography in medical diagnosis.

The evolution of CT, and especially the widespread adoption of MDCT, has led to an exponential growth in the use of CT and in the population radiation dose from medical x-rays. In the 10 years between 1996 and 2006, the number of CT procedures increased almost 3-fold (from 22 to 62 million) in the United States. From 1980 to 2006, the annual population radiation dose from medical procedures increased 7-fold, with CT contributing far more to this increase than any other imaging modality. Today, about 50% of the average radiation dose to individuals in the United States is delivered by medical radiation, much of it from computed tomography.

The technology of CT is formidable, especially since the acquisition of x-ray transmission data is separated from the display of CT images by a complex series of mathematical manipulations. It is tempting for users of computed tomography to assume that the images are correct and to dismiss the need to understand the underlying technology, at least in principle. Without such an understanding, however, users are sometimes unable to determine whether unusual findings in the images are caused by abnormalities in the patient or malfunctions in the technology. Further, a basic understanding of CT technology is necessary if CT is to be employed intelligently, in a manner that reflects a responsible use of radiation, and that is not abusive of fiscal resources.

For CT users who recognize their need to understand the fundamentals of CT, this book is an excellent resource. The author, Dr Mahesh, is an internationally-recognized expert in CT technology and applications, and that expertise is evident in each chapter of the text. Studying this book will provide CT users with not only a fundamental understanding of CT, but also the background necessary to accommodate future technological improvements in CT. Although these improvements cannot be foreseen at this time, it is certainly reasonable to assume that additional improvements will occur; that has been the history of CT since its inception.

Foreword

João A. C. Lima, MD

Scientists and thinkers have speculated that the ability to see in three dimensions played a crucial role in the development of cognitive function among primates and particularly among humans. Humans believe what they see, and commonly use visualization as a means to derive knowledge. Medical science has been no exception. Early efforts to understand the works of the human body through anatomic dissection after the renaissance led to the birth of modern medical knowledge.The discovery and development of x-ray imaging followed by the application of ultrasound, magnetic resonance, and nuclear isotopic technologies to medical imaging have propelled the practice of medicine to the level where it is situated today. Currently, both for diagnostic and therapeutic purposes, medical imaging represents the backbone of sophisticated medical activity in the developed and developing world. In the future, some of the most challenging medical problems such as atherosclerosis, cancer therapeutics and neurologic diagnostics are likely to be understood and brought under control through the use of imaging. Recently, among all imaging methods used for the diagnosis of human disease processes, computed tomography (CT) has played the most important role.

The simplicity of principles, versatility, and power of CT technology are unmatched among imaging modalities. Its importance in daily medical care has transformed medical practice and is likely to produce yet greater paradigm shifts in the near future. CT technological progress has been a consequence of the digital revolution as well as hardware refinement, and its potential for enabling future medical paradigm shifts likely stems from the possibility of enhanced hardware and software integration in the future. This will allow for novel combinations of complex image acquisition and reconstructive approaches with ever more powerful detector systems, gantry mechanics and contrast materials. The breadth and depth of the past technologic achievements and future developments can only be grasped through thorough and comprehensive understanding of CT physics. Such task is the subject of this book.

In the first chapters, the principles of CT and more so of the multiple-row detector CT (MDCT) are explained in a direct and pragmatic style and is complemented by important insights on radiation dose and current strategies to reduce it. The last chapters of the book are equally important and focus on the boundary between the present and the future of MDCT technology. Hybrid imaging systems, advanced methodologies such as CT perfusion and CT fluoroscopy as well as emerging technologies like dual-source CT, whole body and flat-panel CT imaging point to the future, when MDCT may occupy center stage not only in diagnostics but also in image guidance, therapy monitoring and subclinical disease detection.

Finally, it is important that one realizes the landmark importance of this book. It fills a crucial gap for its practical style and comprehensive organization. Moreover, this compilation of knowledge and detailed information on the principles and practice of medical CT technology could not be accomplished by someone who does not live and breathe CT clinical imaging and technologic innovation. The author, Dr. Mahesh, is able to transmit his *hands on* vast experience in the practice of CT and in the teaching of students, residents and faculty colleagues, as well as leading research to discover new ways of enhancing image acquisition, improving study quality and reducing radiation exposure. It is a great privilege to have witnessed both the quantum advances that have recently occurred in CT technology and the author's prominent contributions to their development and implementation in medical practice. This book describes *the state of the art* and points to the bright future of MDCT as a pivotal medical and scientific tool in the quest to augment quality of life and reduce human disease and mortality.

Computed tomography (CT) has been hailed as one of the top five medical innovations in the past four decades according to most medical surveys. The emergence of multiple-row detector CT (MDCT) technology is considered a major evolutionary leap in the field of CT and in the overall field of medical diagnosis. The introduction of MDCT has led to the exponential growth in CT procedures not only in the United States and other developed countries, but also equally across the globe.

The potential benefits of MDCT to medical diagnosis have attracted not only the traditional CT users, but also other physicians and scientists alike. The wide-ranging potential of MDCT technology has led to the introduction of numerous clinical protocols, peaking interest in CT users as to learn the underlying physical principles so as to appreciate the capabilities and limitations of this technology. Clinicians and other CT users have often complained about the lack of a single textbook that can explain, in simple terms, the physics of MDCT technology. Although there are a number of textbooks on MDCT, most have either a short description of the physical principles of MDCT in the midst of a comprehensive textbook on CT, or offer too much detailed description of CT physics with focus on image-reconstruction methods and artifacts.

This book is intended to fill the gap by providing easy-to-read yet comprehensive book on MDCT technology. The primary motivation to write this textbook was to provide an overview of MDCT with a focus on the physical principles of MDCT technology, and the effects of various scan parameters on image quality and radiation dose.

The book contains 12 chapters with more than 150 illustrations and images to explain the physical principles of MDCT. Each chapter presents material in a straightforward manner that is well illustrated and explained.

Chapters 1 and 2 describe the fundamentals of CT principles, inherent advantages of CT images over conventional x-ray images, and provide an overview of various CT generations—from conventional CT to spiral or helical CT all the way up to MDCT.

Chapter 3 discusses the physical principles of MDCT and the distinct differences from previous CT generations. Various detector designs and configurations, from 4-slice to 64-slice technology, are described in this chapter. Illustrations to demonstrate different detector designs utilized in clinical protocols are provided in this chapter. Basic description of the image reconstruction in MDCT is also provided in this chapter. In Chapter 4, various components of MDCT scanner such as CT gantry, the x-ray tube, collimator, and various filters and others are described.

Chapter 5 discusses the various scan parameters that influence image quality and radiation dose. This chapter discusses each scan parameter with illustrations and images to demonstrate the effect on the CT image and radiation dose. The purpose of this chapter is to provide the readers the description and an in-depth analysis of each parameter so that understanding the parameters can help in optimizing respective clinical protocol for better image quality with minimal radiation dose.

Chapter 6 focuses entirely on the principles of cardiac CT physics. Cardiac imaging became feasible with the introduction of MDCT. The field of cardiac CT is growing rapidly and its uniqueness has led to the demand for rapid and fine scanning, and has been the impetus for many technological advances in MDCT. Various data acquisition methods, image reconstruction methods, and scan parameters that influence cardiac CT images are described in this chapter.

Radiation risks are of concern with any x-ray imaging methods. With rapid increase in the number of CT procedures, radiation doses associated with CT scans are attracting even greater attention. For all those associated with CT imaging, understanding the fundamentals of radiation doses is key to fully utilize the benefits of the MDCT technology. Chapter 7 is about radiation dose in CT. Detailed description of the various radiation dose descriptors such as computed tomography dose index (CTDI), dose-length-product (DLP) and effective dose are provided. Also described in this chapter are factors influencing CT dose, with illustrations and images, and tables of doses for various CT procedures.

Chapter 8 describes various radiation dose–reducing strategies developed by the four major MDCT manufacturers. In order to keep the discussion on MDCT impartial, separate sections from each of the four MDCT manufacturers describing their dose–reducing strategies are included in this chapter.

Chapter 9 describes the advantages and principles of dual-modality or hybrid imaging systems. Included in this chapter are the descriptions of fusion imaging of CT with positron emission tomography (PET) and single-photon emission computed tomography (SPECT). In addition to describing principles of PET-CT and SPECT-CT, scan parameters commonly utilized in PET-CT and SPECT-CT are described, along with image artifacts and radiation dose.

MDCT technology is changing so rapidly. To write a book on this subject is like trying to catch a moving bullet. Yet, an attempt is made to cover this technology as much as possible. Chapter 10 discusses recently introduced technologic advances in MDCT such as dual-source CT (DSCT) and 256- to 320-row MDCT technology. Basic principles of CT fluoroscopy and CT perfusion are also discussed in this chapter. Any discussion on MDCT is not complete without discussing quality control and radiation protection issues. It

is even more crucial to understand the importance of radiation safety, especially in the era of increased regulations and concerns about radiation protection for those who work with or around radiation. Chapter 11 describes various aspects of quality control, accreditation, regulations, radiation protection, and radiation shielding related to CT.

Finally, the Chapter 12 examines the future trends in MDCT. It seems that the so-called "slice wars" with regard to the number of slices provided per CT gantry rotation may be reaching a plateau. At the same time, increasing concerns about radiation doses attributable to CT examinations are fueling the efforts to reduce radiation doses and leading to the beginning of the so-called "dose wars." In addition, interests in dual-energy applications, flat panel CT, and the emergence of niche markets of CT with special applications are discussed. A list of references is provided at the end of the book for interested readers to explore further.

This book is intended primarily for radiologists and radiology residents, cardiologists and cardiology residents, and fellows, as well as, radiation technologists and medical physicists. However, other physicians, medical students, scientists, graduate students, and professionals who are dealing with MDCT could also benefit from it. This book can also be used by radiology residents preparing for the physics portion of the American Board of Radiology exam, and by CT technologists preparing for the CT certification exam. This book can be read in its entirety to understand all aspects of MDCT. However, those interested in certain applications of MDCT can choose among the chapters. For example, someone interested in cardiac CT may want to read chapters 3-7 and 10, and those interested in hybrid imaging can select chapters 3, 4, 5, 7 and 9. In short, I hope this book will be used by many medical professionals who use or work with MDCT, and that it will provide a basic understanding of MDCT.

Mahadevappa Mahesh, MS, PhD

Acknowledgements

There are several individuals who have directly or indirectly helped me to understand the MDCT technology and it is indeed a pleasure to express my sincere thanks to all them. Although, it is impossible to acknowledge them all, I have attempted to thank key individuals who made this book possible.

First, I have been very fortunate by being at the right place at the right time. My first job out of graduate school brought me to Johns Hopkins Hospital. It is already been more than 15 years and every day that I enter this great institution, I am overwhelmed by the number of self-motivated colleagues and staff. I am very grateful to be working at Johns Hopkins as it has provided me the opportunity to see the emergence of MDCT technology. I had the rare occasion to work with many versions of MDCT scanners from all major manufacturers, including the very first 4-, 16-, 32-, 64-, 256- and 320-row MDCT scanners and also on the first PET-CT, SPECT-CT, and dual-source CT scanners. This provided me deeper insight into MDCT technology and the development of protocols.

Being the chief physicist at the hospital has provided me a great opportunity to interact with and learn from many of my physician colleagues. Among them I want to specially thank Drs Richard Wahl, Bob Gayler, David Yousem, Stanley Siegelman, David Bluemke, Ihab Kamel, John Carrino, Karen Horton, Frank Bengal, Jane Benson, Hugh Calkins, Edward Shapiro, and David Bush. I also want to express my gratitude to fellow medical physicists, Drs Thomas Beck, Paul Bottomley, and Benjamin Tsui, and to Mr. Michael Harris, for their support and encouragement. I also take this opportunity to thank my Chairman Dr Jonathan Lewin, Martin Donner Professor of Radiology, for his support and encouragement and for creating a very stimulating environment in the department.

Next, I would like to thank all of our CT technologists at Johns Hopkins, including Beatrice Mudge, Jorge Guzman, William Van Daniker, Cassandra Synder, Jefferson Graves, and Jaime Franklin for their assistance in obtaining data and images for this book, and other CT projects. I would also like to acknowledge Deborah Kearney, my quality control staff, and my assistant, Amelia Dimaano and LaVahn Otey for their assistance on this project.

I am honored to have Drs. William R Hendee, Elliot Fishman, and Joao Lima write the foreword for this book. All these years, each of them has greatly influenced and guided me in many ways. Dr William R. Hendee, PhD, a medical physicist, former dean of the graduate school of biomedical sciences at the Medical College of Wisconsin, and author of many books on medical physics, has been my long-time mentor and I am grateful for his foreword. Dr Elliot Fishman, MD, Chief of Body CT, a world-renowned radiologist, and CT expert, was instrumental in my submitting this book proposal to various publishers through his suggestions and encouragement. I have also been very fortunate to have learned many aspects of CT from him. Finally, I would like to thank Dr Joao Lima, MD, a cardiologist and Director of Cardiac CT Imaging at Johns Hopkins. From the onset of cardiac imaging with MDCT, Dr Lima provided me the opportunity to participate in various cardiac CT projects. It is a rare opportunity for a medical physicist to be involved in so many aspects of MDCT from the very beginning. In fact, the interactions and knowledge I gained through research and teaching on this subject finally gave me the confidence to write this book. I am very grateful to all three for writing the foreword, which adds immensely to the value of this book.

I would also like to thank my publishers Lipponcott Williams & Wilkins. I am very grateful for the confidence bestowed on me in signing me to write this book. As we all work under the sharp dagger of due dates, thanks to Ryan Shaw, managing editor for this book project for his constant and timely reminders that led to the completion of this book. I would also like to thank Lisa McAllister, Brian Brown, Kerry Barrett, Angela Panetta, and Ruth Einstein for all their assistance in publishing this book.

I would like also like to acknowledge each of the four major MDCT manufacturers who readily agreed and contributed to the chapter on strategies to reduce CT dose. Among them, I want to sincerely express my gratitude to Drs Sholom Acklesberg and Uri Shreter from GE Healthcare, Drs Christopher Suess and Thomas Flohr from Siemens Medical Systems, and Dr. Richard Mather from Toshiba and Dr. Abraham Cohn from Philips.

Finally, I would like to acknowledge my wife, Vasantha, for her supportive understanding and encouragement. As I spent more and more time on this book, she devoted so much time and energy in taking care of our kids and me. She has been my best friend and critic, and has always kept me focused on the goals. I am grateful for the time she has given up from her own pursuits to allow me to take on many projects, such as this book and others. I also want to acknowledge my children, Ajay and Smitha, for their understanding of the loss of their playtime with me. I warmly recall how they often reminded me to work on this book especially when I interrupted their TV time to watch my shows.

I hope the readers enjoy and benefit from this book as much as I have enjoyed learning about MDCT.

Contents

Introduction

Computed tomography (CT) is one of the top five medical innovations in the last four decades according to most medical surveys. It has proved invaluable as a diagnostic tool for many clinical applications. Since its introduction in 1972, CT has evolved into an essential diagnostic imaging tool for a continually increasing variety of clinical applications. In 1979, Sir Godfrey N. Hounsfield and Alan M. Cormack received the Nobel Prize in medicine for the *development of computer-assisted tomography*. Dramatic improvements in image quality, acquisition speed, and patient throughput have resulted from further technical developments in helical and, more recently, with multiple-row detector technologies. In the early 1990s, the introduction of helical or spiral CT scanners was considered a major breakthrough for CT technology. By mid 1990s, CT technology and its applications were thought to have reached a plateau. However, the introduction of multiple-row detector CT (MDCT) scanner is considered a major evolutionary leap in CT technology.

The introduction of MDCT has led to the exponential growth in the CT procedures not only in the United States or in the developed countries but also equally across the globe. In 2007, the number of CT procedures performed in the United States reached as many as 69 million (Fig. 1.1), with more than 10,000 installed CT scanners. The explosion of CT procedures in United States alone exceeds 10% annually from the time MDCT technology became available. With newer applications getting acceptance, the

trend for future growth in CT is even stronger. In fact, the meteoric rise in the acceptance of MDCT technology is self-evident in the increasing dominance of this technology (Fig. 1.2, Table 1.1). According to a survey conducted in 2007, more than 80% of all CT scanners installed in the United States were MDCT scanners (Fig. 1.3), which is a rapid growth for a technology that became available only around the turn of the century (four-slice MDCT scanner became commercially available only around 1998).

If one considers the evolution of the technology as a progression toward optimizing the information content of radiographic images and extending the method to three dimensions, i.e., to achieve isotropic resolution (the holy grail of medical imaging), then the inherent advantages of MDCT technology that make it possible not only to scan at submillimeter spatial resolution but also to achieve high temporal resolution with shorter scan times have lead to the development of a true three-dimensional imaging tool. MDCT technology has led to the development of many new clinical applications and clinical protocols and has resulted in a diverse group of users. Its inherent ease of use and its capability to yield high-quality images all have contributed to the proliferation of MDCT technology throughout the hospital and not confined to the radiology department, as in the past. With ever-expanding applications with MDCT and the radiation dose associated with various protocols, it becomes important to understand the principles of this technology, along with the interdependency of the various

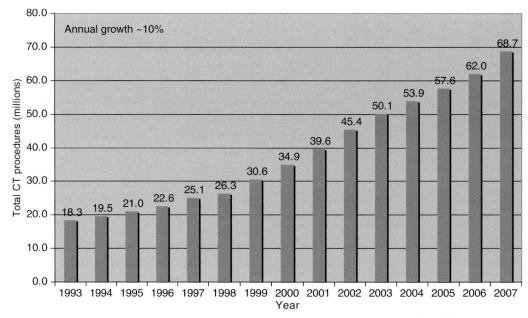

Figure 1.1. Number of CT procedures performed in the United States for the period of 1993–2007. Annual growth is approximately 10%.

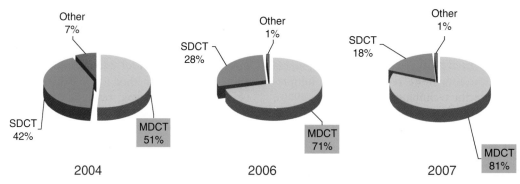

Figure 1.2. MDCT growth in United States as percent CT scanners in clinical use.

Table 1.1	Percent growth of MDCT scanners in clinical use in United States		
Survey year	**2004**	**2006**	**2007**
Total CT installed in United States	9,380	10,110	10,300
MDCT, %	**51**	**71**	**81**
SDCT, %	42	28	18
Other, %	7	1	1

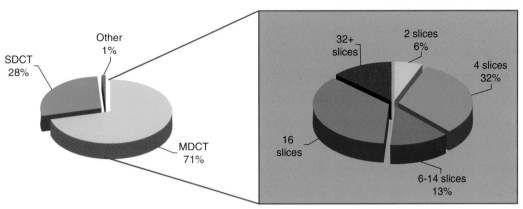

Figure 1.3. MDCT distribution based on number of slices in United States during 2006.

scan parameters on image quality and radiation dose. This book is an attempt to explore various aspects of MDCT technology, including multiple-row detector designs (i.e., 4- to 64-row MDCT), scan parameters, cardiac CT, hybrid CT (positron emission tomography [PET]-CT and single-photon emission computed tomography [SPECT]-CT), advanced technologies such as dual-source CT and 320-row MDCT, and radiation dose.

Conventional, Spiral, and Electron Beam CT: Background

In conventional x-ray imaging, a uniform x-ray beam is directed at the patient, and it exits the opposite surface encoded with intensity variations as the result of differential attenuation of x-rays along different paths through the patient. The intensity-encoded pattern is then recorded on a two-dimensional surface (i.e., the radiographic image receptor). Radiographic systems have themselves evolved considerably, and current imaging systems promise spatial resolution in excess of five line-pairs per millimeter with acquisition times in the tens to hundreds of milliseconds. However, radiographic image quality has some limitations. Film-based systems are nonlinear, and the ability to discriminate small tissue differences is largely limited by poor scatter discrimination. One major problem that limits clinical usefulness is the fact that radiographic images superimpose three-dimensional anatomy onto a two-dimensional surface (Fig. 2.1). Historically, much of the training that radiologists have received has been dedicated to mentally reconstructing the three-dimensional anatomical relationships from one or more radiographic projections with overlapping anatomy to determine whether altered patterns signal the presence of disease.

One might state that the ideal x-ray imaging system would be able to combine the attributes of conventional radiography but also solve some of its limitations. Thus, such a system would be able to produce images with spatial resolution on the order of five line-pairs per millimeter and acquisition times of a few hundred milliseconds sufficient to freeze physiologic motion. In addition, the ideal system would respond linearly over a wide range, would exclude contrast-robbing scatter, and provide three-dimensional information free of superimposing tissues with equal resolution throughout (isotropic resolution). Even the earliest computed tomography (CT) scanners progressed toward this goal. Early scanners obtained images of transverse sections through the body, thus avoiding the problem of superimposed tissues. The narrow beam geometry and special collimation effectively eliminated scatter, thus greatly improving the contrast detectability over radiographic methods. With respect to spatial resolution and acquisition times, however, early scanners had a very long way to go to achieve near radiographic performance in three dimensions.

Computed Tomography

CT is fundamentally a method for acquiring and reconstructing an image of a thin cross section of an object. It differs from conventional projection in two significant ways: CT forms a cross-sectional image, eliminating the superimposition of structures that occurs in plane film imaging because of compression of three-dimensional body structures onto the two-dimensional recording system and, second, the sensitivity of CT to subtle differences in x-ray attenuation is at least a factor of 10 greater than normally achieved by film screen recording systems because of the virtual elimination of scatter (Fig. 2.2). It is based on measurements of x-ray attenuation through the section using many different projections.

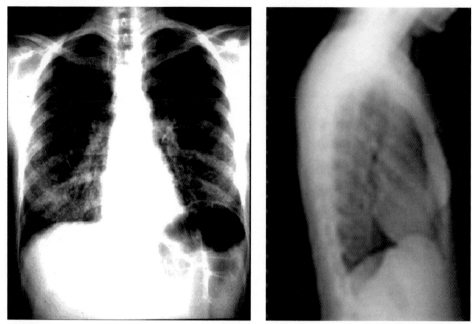

Figure 2.1. Radiographs of chest region show limitation for diagnosis with tissue superimposition. Radiographs are two-dimensional maps of three-dimensional anatomy.

Basic Principles of CT

Fundamentally, a CT scanner makes many measurements of attenuation through the plane of a finite thickness cross section of the body. The system uses that data to reconstruct a digital image of the cross section where each pixel in the image represents a measurement of the mean attenuation of a box-like element (voxel) extending through the thickness of the section (Fig. 2.3).

An attenuation measurement quantifies the fraction of radiation removed in passing through a given amount of a specific material of thickness, Δx, as shown in Figure 2.4A. Attenuation is expressed as:

$$I_t = I_o e^{-\mu \Delta x} \qquad (1)$$

where, I_t and I_o are the x-ray intensities measured with and without the material in the x-ray beam path, respectively, and μ is the linear

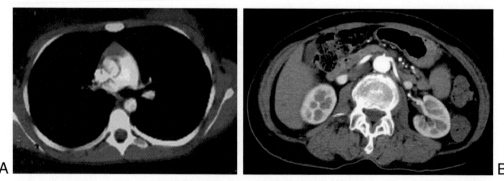

Figure 2.2. CT provide two-dimensional images of approximately two-dimensional cross-sectional slices of the body from multiple projections. **A:** Chest CT image. **B:** Abdominal CT image

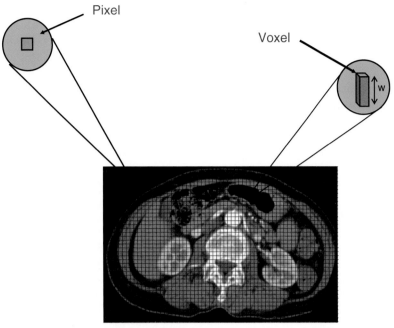

Figure 2.3. The CT image is composed of *pixels* (picture elements). Each pixel on the image represents the average x-ray attenuation in a small volume *(voxel)* extending through the tissue slice. (Pixel size is exaggerated and, in a real CT image, all tissues within a single pixel would have the same shade of gray.) (From Mahesh M. Search for Isotropic Resolution in CT from conventional through multiple-row detector. *Radio-Graphics* 2002;22:949–962, with permission).

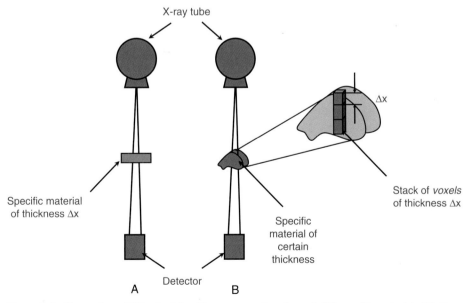

Figure 2.4. Illustration of CT principles. X-ray attenuation through **(A)** specific material of finite thickness (Δx) (refer to Eq. 1) and **(B)** material considered as stack of voxels with each voxel of finite thickness (Δx) (refer to Eq. 2) (From Mahesh M. Search for isotropic resolution in CT from conventional through multiple-row detector. *RadioGraphics* 2002;22:949–962, 2002 with permission.)

attenuation coefficient of the specific material. To illustrate CT principles, any material can be considered as a stack of voxels along the beam path (Fig. 2.4B). Each attenuation measurement is called a *ray sum* because attenuation along a specific straight-line path through the patient from the tube focal spot to a detector is the sum of the individual attenuations of all materials along the path. Assuming that the ray path through the tissue is broken up into incremental voxel thicknesses Δx, the transmitted intensity is given by:

$$I_t = I_o e^{-\sum_{i=1}^{k} \mu_i \Delta x} \qquad (2)$$

Expressed as the natural logarithm (ln):

$$\ln\left[\frac{I_o}{I_t}\right] = \sum_{i=1}^{k} \mu_i \Delta x \qquad (3)$$

The image reconstruction process derives the average attenuation coefficient (μ) values for each voxel in the cross section using many rays from many different rotational angles around the cross section. The specific attenuation of a voxel (μ) increases with the density and the atomic numbers of tissues averaged through the volume of the voxel and decreases with increasing x-ray energy.

Mathematically, the attenuation (μ) value for each voxel could be solved algebraically with a very large number of simultaneous equations using all ray sums that intersect the voxel. However, a much more elegant and simpler method, called *filtered back-projection*, was used in the early CT scanners and remains in use today. Rays are collected in sets called *projections* that are made across the patient in a particular direction through the section plane. There may be from 500 to 1000 or more rays in a single projection. To reconstruct the image from the ray measurements, each voxel must be viewed from multiple different directions. A complete data set requires many projections at fine rotational intervals of 1 degree or less around the cross section. Back projection effectively reverses the attenuation process by adding the attenuation value of each ray in each projection back through the reconstruction matrix. Because this process generates a blurred image, the data from each projection are mathematically altered (filtered) before back projection, eliminating the intrinsic blurring effect. There are number of advanced reconstruction techniques discussed in later chapters.

As a final process, the individual voxel attenuation values are scaled to more convenient integers and normalized to voxel values containing water (μ_w). CT numbers are computed as:

$$CT\# = K\left[\frac{\mu_m - \mu_w}{\mu_w}\right] \qquad (4)$$

where, μ_m is the measured attenuation of the material in the voxel and K (1000) is the scaling factor. The attenuation coefficient of water is obtained during calibration of the CT machine. Voxels containing materials that attenuate more than water, for example, muscle tissue, liver, and bone, have positive CT numbers, whereas materials with less attenuation than water, such as lung or adipose tissues, have negative CT numbers. With the exception of water and air, the CT numbers for a given material will vary with changes in the x-ray tube potential and from manufacturer to manufacturer.

Historical Developments

In 1979, Sir Godfrey N. Hounsfield (Fig. 2.5) and Alan M. Cormack were awarded the Nobel Prize in medicine for the development of computer-assisted tomography. The mathematical principles of image reconstruction date earlier to Radon in 1917. A variety of CT geometries have been developed to acquire the x-ray transmission data for image reconstruction. These geometries are commonly called "generations" and remain useful in differentiating scanner designs.

CT Generations

First-Generation CT Scanners. The EMI Mark I scanner, the first commercial scanner invented by Hounsfield, was introduced in 1973. This scanner acquired data with an x-ray beam collimated to a narrow "pencil" beam directed to a single detector on the other side of the patient;

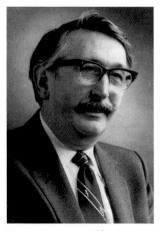
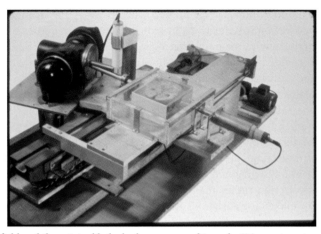

Figure 2.5. Sir Godfrey N. Housefield and the original lathe bed scanner used in early CT experiments.

the detector and the beam were aligned in a scanning frame. A single projection was acquired by moving the tube and detector in a straight-line motion (translation) on opposite sides of the patient (Fig. 2.6). To acquire the next projection, the frame rotated 1 degree then translated in the other direction. This process of translation and rotation was repeated until 180 projections were obtained. The earliest versions required about 4.5 minutes for a single scan and thus were restricted to regions where patient motion could be controlled (head). Because the procedures consisted of a series of scans, the procedure time was reduced somewhat by using two detectors so that two parallel sections were acquired in one scan. Although contrast resolution of internal structures was unprecedented, the images had poor spatial resolution (on the order of 3 mm for a field of view of 25 cm and 80 × 80 matrix) and very poor z-axis resolution (~13 mm slice thickness) (Fig. 2.7).

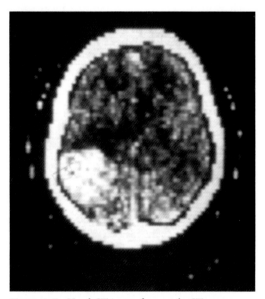

Figure 2.7. Head CT image from early CT scanner (scan plane resolution is of the order of 3 mm for a field of view of 25 cm with 80 × 80 matrix and z-axis resolution of the order of approximately 13 mm). (From Mahesh M. Search for isotropic resolution in CT from conventional through multiple-row detector. *RadioGraphics* 2002;22:949–962, with permission.)

Figure 2.6. Sketch of the first-generation CT scanner that used parallel x-ray beam with translate-rotate motion to acquire data. (From Mahesh M. Search for isotropic resolution in CT from conventional through multiple-row detector. *RadioGraphics* 2002;22:949–962, with permission.)

Second-Generation CT Scanners. The main impetus for improvement was in reducing scan time ultimately to the point that regions in the trunk could be imaged. By adding detectors angularly displaced, several projections could be obtained in a single translation. For example, one early design used three detectors each displaced by 1 degree. Because each detector viewed the x-ray tube at a different angle, a single translation produced three projections. Hence, the system could rotate 3 degrees to the next projection rather than 1 degree and had only to make 60 translations instead of 180 to acquire a complete slice (Fig. 2.8). Scan times were reduced by a factor of three. Designs of this type had up to 53 detectors and were ultimately fast enough (tens of seconds) to permit acquisition during a single breath-hold; thus, they were the first designs to permit scans of the trunk of the body. Because rotating anode tubes could not withstand the wear and tear of rotate–translate motion, this design required a relatively low-output stationary anode x-ray tube. The power limits of stationary anodes for efficient heat dissipation were improved somewhat with the use of asymmetrical focal spots (smaller in scan plane than in z-axis direction), but this change resulted in greater radiation doses as the result of poor beam restriction to

the scan plane. Nevertheless, these scanners required slower scan speeds to obtain adequate x-ray flux at the detectors when scanning thicker patients or body parts.

Third-Generation CT Scanners. Designers realized that if a pure rotational scanning motion could be used, then it would be possible to use higher-power, rotating anode x-ray tubes and, thus, improve scan speeds on thicker body parts. One of the first designs to do so was the so-called third-generation or rotate–rotate geometry. In these scanners, the x-ray tube is collimated to a wide fan-shaped x-ray beam and directed toward an arc-shaped row of detectors. During scanning, the tube and detector array rotate around the patient (Fig. 2.9), and different projections are obtained during rotation by pulsing the x-ray source or by sampling the detectors at a very high rate. The number of detectors varied from 300 in early versions to 700 or so in modern scanners. Because the slam-bang translation motion was replaced with smooth rotational motion, greater output rotating anode x-ray tubes could be used and greatly reduced scan times. One aspect of this geometry is that rays in a single projection are divergent

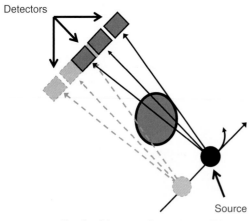

Figure 2.8. Sketch of the second-generation CT scanner with translate-rotation motion to acquire data. From Mahesh M. Search for isotropic resolution in CT from conventional through multiple-row detector. *RadioGraphics* 2002;22:949–962, with permission.)

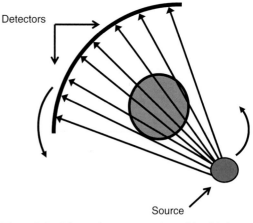

Figure 2.9. Schematic representation of the third-generation CT scanner, which acquires data by rotating both the x-ray source with a wide fan beam geometry and detectors around the patient and, hence, the geometry is called *rotate–rotate* motion. From Mahesh M. Search for isotropic resolution in CT from conventional through multiple-row detector. *RadioGraphics* 2002;22:949–962, with permission.)

rather than parallel to each other as in earlier designs. Beam divergence required some modification of reconstruction algorithms, and sampling considerations required scanning an additional arc of one fan angle beyond 180°, although most scanners rotate 360° for each scan. All current CT scanners are based on modifications of this design. Typical scan times are on the order of a few seconds or less and recent versions are capable of subsecond scan times.

Fourth-Generation CT Scanners. This design evolved nearly simultaneously with third generation scanners and also eliminated translate-rotate motion. In this case, only the source rotates within a stationary ring of detectors (Fig. 2.10). The x-ray tube is positioned to rotate about the patient within the space between the patient and the outer detector ring. One clever version, which is no longer produced, moved the x-ray tube out of the detector ring and tilted the ring out of the x-ray beam in a wobbling (nutation) motion as the tube rotated.

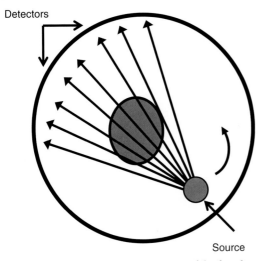

Detectors

Source

Figure 2.10. Schematic representation of the fourth-generation CT scanner; which uses a stationary ring of detectors positioned around the patient. Only the x-ray source rotates, using wide fan beam geometry, whereas the detectors are stationary and hence called *rotate-stationary* motion. From Mahesh M. Search for isotropic resolution in CT from conventional through multiple-row detector. *RadioGraphics* 2002;22:949–962, with permission.)

This design permitted a smaller detector ring with fewer detectors for a similar level of performance. Early fourth-generation scanners had some 600 detectors and later versions up to 4800. Within the same time period, scan times of fourth-generation designs were comparable with those of third-generation scanners. One limitation of fourth-generation designs is their less efficient use of detectors because less than one-fourth is used at any point during scanning. These scanners also are more susceptible to scatter artifacts than third-generation types because they cannot use antiscatter collimators. CT scanners of this design are no longer commercially available.

Until around 1990, CT technology had evolved to deliver scan plane resolutions of 1 to 2 line pairs per millimeter, but z-axis resolution remained poor and interscan delay was problematic because of the stop–start action necessary for table translation and for cable unwinding, which resulted in longer examination times. The z-axis resolution was limited by the choice of slice thickness, which ranged from 1 to 10 mm. For thicker slices, the partial volume averaging between different tissues led to partial volume artifacts. These artifacts were reduced to some extent by scanning thinner slices. Also, conventional method of slice-by-slice acquisition produced misregistration of lesions between sections as the result of involuntary motion of anatomy in subsequent breath-holds between scans. It was soon realized that if multiple sections could be acquired in a single breath-hold, a considerable improvement in the ability to image lesions in regions susceptible to physiologic motion could result. However, this required some technological advances, which led to the development of helical CT scanners.

Principles of Helical CT Scanners

The development of helical or spiral CT around 1990 was a truly revolutionary advancement in CT scanning that finally allowed true three-dimensional image acquisition within a single patient breath-hold. The technique involves the continuous acquisition of projection data through a three-dimensional volume of tissue

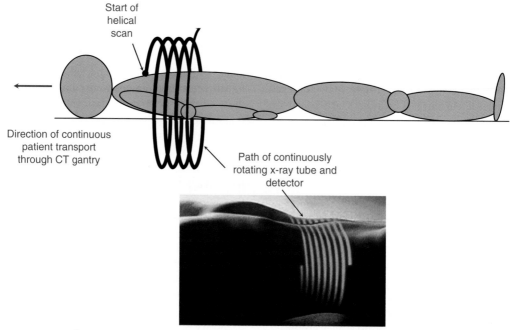

Start of
helical
scan

Direction of continuous
patient transport
through CT gantry

Path of continuously
rotating x-ray tube and
detector

Figure 2.11. Illustration of the principles of helical CT. As the patient is transported through the gantry, the x-ray tube traces a spiral/helical path around the patient, acquiring data as it rotates.

by continuous rotation of the x-ray tube and detectors and simultaneous translation of the patient through the gantry opening (Fig. 2.11). Three technological developments were required: slip-ring gantry designs, very high power x-ray tubes, and interpolation algorithms to handle the noncoplanar projection data.

Slip-Ring Technology. Slip rings are electromechanical devices consisting of circular electrical conductive rings and brushes that transmit electrical energy across a moving interface. All power and control signals from the stationary parts of the scanner system are communicated to the rotating frame through the slip ring. The slip-ring design consists of sets of parallel conductive rings concentric to the gantry axis that connects to the tube, detectors and control circuits by sliding contractors (Fig. 2.12). These *sliding contractors* allow the scan frame to rotate continuously with no need to stop between rotations to rewind system cables. This engineering advancement resulted initially from a desire to reduce interscan delay and improve throughput. However, reduced interscan delay

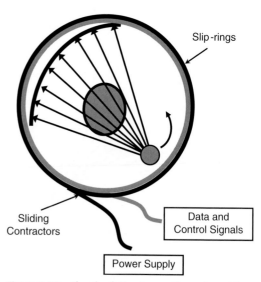

Slip-rings

Sliding
Contractors

Data and
Control Signals

Power Supply

Figure 2.12. Sketch of slip-ring configuration with sliding contractors to permit continuous rotation of x-ray tube and detectors while maintaining electrical contact with stationary components. From Mahesh M. Search for isotropic resolution in CT from conventional through multiple-row detector. *Radio-Graphics* 2002;22:949–962, with permission.)

increased the thermal demands on the x-ray tube; hence, tubes with much greater thermal capacities were required to withstand continuous operation over multiple rotations.

High-Power X-Ray Tubes. Compared with any other diagnostic x-ray application, CT x-ray tubes are subjected to far greater thermal loads. In early CT scanners, such as in first- and second-generation ones, stationary anode x-ray tubes were used because the long scan times meant the instantaneous power level was low. Long scan times also allowed for heat dissipation. Shorter scan times in later versions of CT scanners required high-power x-ray tube and use of oil-cooled rotating anodes for efficient thermal dissipation. Heat storage capacities varied from 1 to 3 million heat units (MHU) in early third-generation CT scanners. The introduction of helical CT with continuous scanner rotation placed new demands on x-ray tubes. Several technical advances in component design have been made to achieve these power levels and address the problems of target temperature, heat storage, and dissipation. Because many of the engineering changes increase the mass of the tube, much of the design effort also was dedicated to reduce the mass to better withstand increasing gantry rotational rates required by ever faster scan times. Modern CT tubes have capacities of 5–8 MHU that can basically run continuously without the need to stop for cooling.

Interpolation Algorithms. Conventional scanners stepped the patient through the gantry to provide a series of contiguous sections, but it was soon realized that if acquisition could be performed with continuous table motion, then a much more satisfactory result would be obtained. The problem with continuous tube and table motion was that projections precessed in a helical motion around the patient and did not lie in a single plane, meaning that conventional reconstruction algorithms could not work. Prof. Willi Kallendar (Fig. 2.13) is credited with solving this problem by developing interpolation methods to generate projections in a single plane so that conventional back projections could be used. There were several important benefits to this development. First, the reconstruction planes could

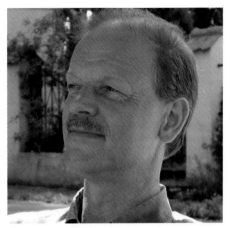

Figure 2.13. Prof. Willi Kalendar credited for developing helical CT.

be placed in any arbitrary position along the scanned volume encompassed by the table traverse during multiple rotations. This meant that sections could be overlapping along the scan axis, thus greatly improving data sampling and making three-dimensional reconstructions practical. Second, because images can be acquired in a single breath-hold, the three-dimensional reconstructions are free of the misregistration artifacts caused by involuntary motion that bedevil conventional CT. True three-dimensional volumes could be acquired that can be viewed in any perspective, making the promise of true three-dimensional radiography a practical reality. A final benefit was that because overlapping slices were generated by mathematical methods rather than overlapping x-ray beams, the improved z-axis sampling was obtained without a radiation dose penalty to the patient. A number of advanced interpolation algorithms have been developed with differing effects on image quality and can be found in most image reconstruction books.

Capabilities of Single-Row Detector Helical CT

With the advent of helical CT, considerable progress was attained on the road toward three-dimensional radiography. An example of a three-dimensional reconstruction from single-row helical computed tomography (SDCT) scanning is shown in Figure 2.14. Complete

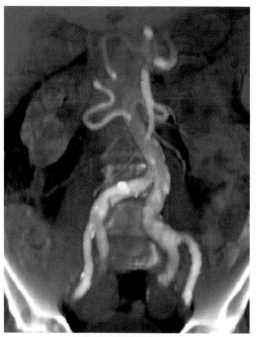

Figure 2.14. Three-dimensional reconstructed images from single-row detector helical CT data. (From Elliot Fishman, MD, Johns Hopkins Hospital, Baltimore, MD, with permission.)

scans, the table motion causes displacement of the fan-beam projections along the z-axis; the relative displacement is a function of the table speed and the beam width. The ratio of table displacement per 360-degree rotation to section thickness is termed pitch, an important dimensionless quantity with implications for patient dose and image quality (discussed in more detail in later Chapter 5). Although the z-axis resolution for helical CT images far exceeds that of conventional CT images, still the type of interpolation algorithm and pitch affects the overall image quality. The slice sensitivity profiles of helical CT images are different compared with conventional CT images, which are influenced by the type of interpolation algorithm and selected pitch. Also, with a single-row of detectors in the longitudinal direction, the scan volume covered per gantry rotation is limited to single-slice dimension. Continued scanner development on the road to a three-dimensional radiograph demanded further progress and led to the development of multiple-row detector CT (MDCT) scanners.

Electron Beam CT

As third- and fourth-generation conventional CT scanners became popular by early 1980s, many investigators attempted imaging the most challenging organ, the heart. However, by using the scanners then available, they achieved little success. Imaging the heart is a challenge because of the rapid motion, variation in motion caused by variable heart rates, the location of the heart itself, and also the vessels of variable sizes. With many technical limitations such as longer scan times, x-ray tube heating, and others, it was not possible to image moving heart without plagued with motion artifacts. In the early 1980s Boyd and colleagues designed and built the very first ultrafast CT scanner, which is familiarly known as *electron beam CT* (EBCT) which made CT imaging of heart and coronary arteries practical. The technology differed from conventional CT system with the immovable x-ray source that enabled fast data acquisition in the order of 50 to 100 milliseconds. After the arrival of MDCT scanners, the use of EBCT became scarce and eventually from 2003 onwards, EBCT became unavailable for commercial use. For interest of

organs could be scanned in approximately 30–40 seconds. In addition, artifacts caused by patient motion and tissue misregistration caused by involuntary motion were virtually eliminated. It became possible to generate slices in any arbitrary plane through the scanned volume.

Significant improvements in z-axis resolution were achieved as the result of improved sampling because slices could be reconstructed at fine intervals less than the section width along the z-axis. Near-isotropic resolution could be obtained with the thinnest (~1 mm) section widths at a pitch of one, but this could only be performed over relatively short lengths because of tube and breath-hold limitations. Higher power tubes capable of longer continuous operation coupled with faster rotation speeds could scan larger lengths by higher resolution.

The practical limit on such brute force approaches, however, became the length of time a sick patient could reliably hold his or her breath, a time that works out to be no longer than 30 seconds on average. During helical

understanding the background of CT, a brief description of this technology is provided here.

Principles of Electron Beam CT. EBCT used an electron gun and stationary rings of tungsten "targets" rather than a stationary x-ray tube to generate x-rays, thus permitting very rapid scanning times (Fig. 2.15). X-rays were produced by sweeping a highly focused electron beam around the semicircular tungsten targets The 210-degree target ring centered below the patient at a radius of 90 cm from scanner iso-center acted as the source for x-ray production. A stationary detector ring was centered above the patient and formed a 216-degree arc

opposite the target ring. The x-rays produced around the tungsten ring are captured by the ring of detectors, which were then transmitted to computers for reconstruction. The detector ring comprised two detector arrays, one having nearly half of detector elements than the other. Single or multiple slices were obtained by focusing electron beams on single or multiple target rings. Serial axial images were obtained in 50 to 100 ms with a thickness of 3 to 6 mm. A total of 30 to 40 adjacent axial scans usually are obtained during one to two breath-holding sequences and are triggered by the electrocardiographic signal set to certain portion of the R-R interval, near end diastole before atrial

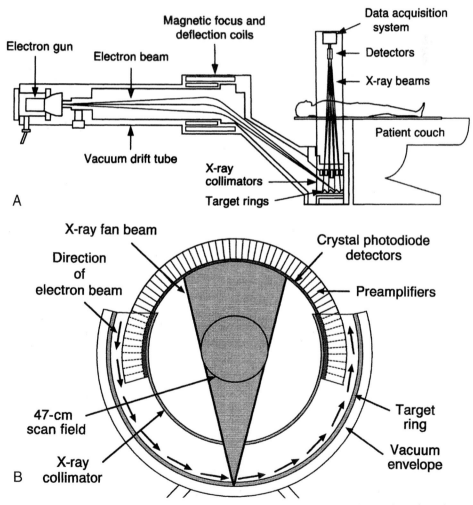

Figure 2.15. Illustration of an electron beam CT scanner. (From McCollough RL. The technical design and performance of ultrafast computer tomography. *Radiol Clin North Am* 1994;21:521, with permission.)

contraction. The rapid image acquisition time virtually eliminates motion artifact related to cardiac contraction.

The main strength of EBCT technology is its ability to acquire cross-sectional x-ray images in times as short as 50 or 100 ms, which is unmatched even by the current CT system stand-ards. EBCT technology is technically complex and, thus, EBCT remained a dedicated scanner for cardiac imaging only. On the other hand, the MDCT systems are less complex and widely available and many view cardiac protocols have been developed for these systems which ulti-mately led to the commercial demise of EBCT.

3

Multiple-Row Detector Computed Tomography

In the early 1990s, the introduction of helical or spiral computed tomography (CT) scanners was considered a major breakthrough for CT technology. By mid 1990s, CT technology and its applications were thought to reach a plateau. However, the introduction of multiple-row detector CT scanner (MDCT) is considered a major evolutionary leap in CT technology. It all started with one vendor's (Elscint–Picker–Philips) introduction of a dual-row detector spiral CT scanner in mid-1990s. Elscint introduced a *twin CT* with the capability to produce dual scans per x-ray tube gantry rotation. In this scanner, the detector was split into two columns that enabled one to obtain dual scans. Actually, the very first CT introduced by Hounsfield, back in 1974, had the capability to produce two scans. By late 1998, all major CT manufacturers launched MDCT scanners capable of at least four slices per x-ray tube rotation. This technology has been called by many names, including MDCT, multislice CT, multidetector CT, and volume CT. **Multiple-row detector CT** or **MDCT** is the term used throughout this textbook for describing this technology.

Until the arrival of MDCT scanners, all CT scanners consist of multiple detector elements in the scan plane or x–y plane but only had one row of detectors in the longitudinal or z-axis. There are typically 700 to 900 detectors in the axial plane (x–y plane). This number of detectors forms the range of the arc of the x-ray beam as discussed in Chapter 2 in the section "Third-Generation Computed Tomography Scanners." The principal difference between single- and multiple-row detector CT scanners is illustrated in Figure 3.1. In the Figure 3.1, a side view of detector schematics demonstrates that the number of rows of detector is increased from one to eight. Basically, while maintaining same number of detectors in the x-ray plane, the number of rows of detectors is increased in z-direction, providing multiple-row detectors in z-direction with capability to yield multiple scans per single rotation of x-ray tube in the CT gantry.

The total number of detector elements depends upon the number of detector elements in x-ray plane (700–900) times the number of rows of detectors (2 to 4, 8, 16, or 64 rows), yielding total detector elements in the range of 1400–60,000. If the detector elements are viewed from the x-ray portal side, it appears more like a square mosaic. Figure 3.2 shows photographs of the detector elements for both a single-row detector CT (SDCT) and MDCT. The important component in MDCT scanner is the data acquisition systems (DAS). These DAS channels determine the actual number of multiple rows that are used to acquire data that ultimately yield multiple slices during data acquisition.

The basic idea actually dates to the very first EMI Mark I scanner, which had two parallel detectors and acquired two slices simultaneously. The first helical scanner to use this idea, the Elscint CT Twin, was launched in the mid-1990s. Although the original company was bought out—sold or gobbled up by large company—few manufacturers still offer such dual-slice systems in their product line. This design was so superior to single-row designs that all scanner manufacturers went back to the drawing

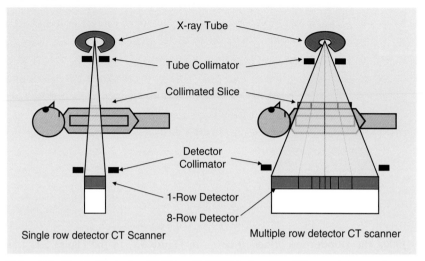

Figure 3.1. Sketch illustrating SDCT and MDCT design. The difference between the two is the presence of multiple-row detectors in the longitudinal direction, with MDCT yielding multiple slices for single gantry rotation.

board. By late 1998, all major CT manufacturers launched multiple-row detector CT scanners capable of at least four slices per rotation. The arrangement of detectors along the z-axis and the widths of the available slices vary between the systems.

As shown in the Figure 3.1, except for the number of detector-rows and the width of the x-ray beam, everything else is similar between SDCT and MDCT. The number of slices obtained per x-ray tube rotation around the patient is defined at the patient plane (isocenter). In SDCT designs, scan volume can be increased with a wider section width, at the expense of poorer z-axis resolution, whereas z-axis resolution can be preserved or even

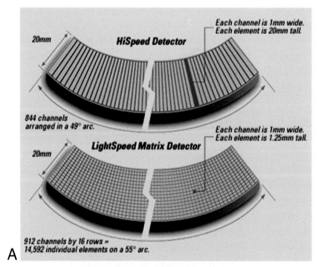

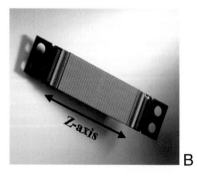

*GE LightSpeed, GE Medical Systems   *Aquillion 16, Toshiba Medical System

Figure 3.2. MDCT detectors. **A:** Photograph of detector elements used in SDCT (HiSpeed detector) and MDCT (LightSpeed matrix detector) system (from GE Health care, Waukesha, WI, with permission). **B:** Photograph of detector elements used in multiple-row detector CT (Aquillion 16) scanner (from Toshiba Medical Systems, Nasu, Japan, with permission).

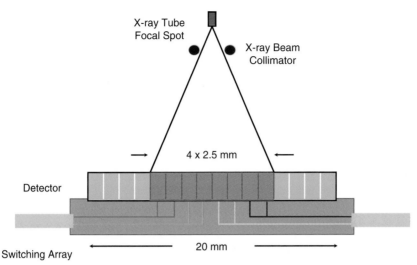

Figure 3.3. Illustration of detector configuration for 4 × 2.5 mm. Shown here is the detector configuration in which data from two individual detector elements are combined and captured by a single DAS channel. The total x-ray beam width is 10 mm (4 × 2.25 mm) and the data acquired is then utilized in reconstructing four slices. The minimum slice thickness that can be obtained with this configuration is 2.5 mm or greater.

improved in multiple-row detector designs. For example, if a 10-mm collimation were divided into four 2.5-mm detectors, the same scan length could be obtained in the same time but with a z-axis resolution improved from 10 mm to 2.5 mm (Fig. 3.3). Similarly, an even more improved spatial resolution can be obtained for the same scan time with half of scan length with a configuration of four 1.25-mm detectors (Fig. 3.4). In another example, a multiple-row detector

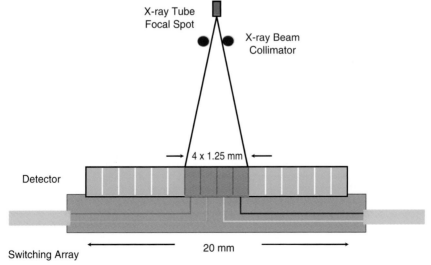

Figure 3.4. Illustration of detector configuration for 4 × 1.25 mm. Shown here is the detector configuration in which each of the four DAS channels collect data from four individual detector elements only. The total x-ray beam width is 5 mm (4 × 1.25 mm) and can be modified with different detector configuration. Data acquired in this way is used to reconstruct individual slices. The minimum slice thickness that can be obtained with this configuration is 1.25 mm or greater.

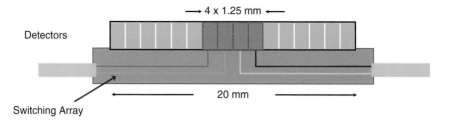

4-section scanners collect
4 simultaneous channels of data

Figure 3.5. Illustrate how the detector elements are used in MDCT scanner. Although the detector array shown in this figure consists of 16 individual detector elements, the number of DAS channels available is four, which ultimately determines the number of slices available for each gantry rotation.

scanner with four detectors of 5 mm each in dimension yielding a beam width of 20 mm reduces the scan time by a factor of 4 for the same z-axis resolution. By increasing the number of CT scanner rows, data acquisition capability dramatically increases while greatly improving the efficiency of x-ray tubes. Further developments in scanner rotational speeds, such as the gantry rotation time decreased from 1 s to less than 0.3 s (300 ms) and increased tube outputs have made isotropic resolution a practical possibility with even greater improvements on the horizon.

In the first-generation MDCT scanners, the common element among all major CT vendors was that only four slices were obtained simultaneously for each gantry rotations. Although there were greater numbers of detector elements

(>4), the number of simultaneous slices (i.e., 4) obtained still was limited by the number of data acquisition system channels (i.e., DAS channels) (Fig. 3.5).

The types of multiple-row detector array designs can be broadly classified into three types: *uniform or matrix array detectors, non-uniform or adaptive array detectors, and hybrid array detectors.* Figure 3.6 illustrates different multiple-row detector array configurations from several vendors. The width of each detector row described to follow is not given as its actual physical width but instead as the width of the corresponding x-ray beam at the center of the scan field. The physical width of the detector may be twice this large, depending on the geometry of the CT scanner and also the distance from center of the scan field to the actual detector

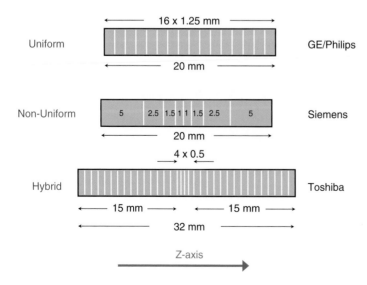

Figure 3.6. Detector element arrays designs used in the first-generation MDCT scanners. Although each of the detector designs consisted of large number of individual detector elements, the maximum number of slices that could be obtained per gantry rotation was four. The number of slices that could be obtained per gantry rotation was limited by the available number of DAS channels.

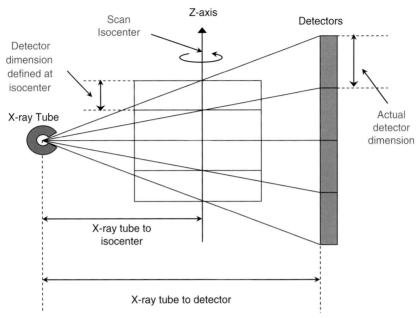

Figure 3.7. Actual detector dimension versus specified detector dimension at isocenter. In MDCT, the detector dimensions such as 4 × 1.25 mm or 4 × 5 mm are defined at the isocenter of the CT gantry. In reality, the actual detector dimensions are larger than the specified detector dimension and depend on the scanner geometry.

(Fig. 3.7). For example, for the scanner geometry of source to detector distance of 1035 mm and source to center of scan field of 570 mm, the detector element's width, defined as 0.5 mm on the patient surface, is actually 0.9 mm wide and, similarly, a detector width of 1 mm is 1.82 mm in actual physical width. Because the CT users ultimately are interested in the slice thickness and not in the physical dimensions of the detectors, the detector widths are defined at the center of the scan field. Also, because it is convenient to understand detector arrays from various manufacturers irrespective of the scanner geometry, the widths of each detector row is defined at the isocenter of the CT gantry.

Uniform or Matrix Array Detectors. In this type of detector array design, several solid-state small detectors of the same dimension are arranged in rows of identical thickness (For example, 16 rows of 1.25 mm) (Fig. 3.8). The image acquired depends on the x-ray beam width, selection of detector rows, and how the two are coupled. It is possible to acquire four simultaneous slices of 1.25 mm each or to increase

the slice thickness by coupling rows of detectors, for example, coupling two, three, and four detector rows together to obtain four slices of 2.5, 3.75, and 5 mm, respectively. In case of 4 × 1.25-mm acquisition, four signals are collected from four 1.25-mm detector rows. However, for a 4 × 2.5-mm configuration, the four signals are collected from eight 1.25-mm detector rows with two detector rows contributing to each signal. Similarly, one could obtain 4 × 2.5 mm, 4 × 3.75 mm, and 4 × 5 mm to yield slices of 2.5 mm, 3.75 mm, and 5 mm, respectively. In each of these cases, multiple rows of detectors contributed to signals yielding thicker slices (Table 3.1). One of the four major MDCT vendors, GE (GE Healthcare, Waukesha, WI) introduced this detector array design.

Nonuniform or Variable Array Detectors. In this type of detector array, the detector width gradually increases in thickness as it moves away from the center of axis of rotation (Fig. 3.9). The two detector rows in the center of the array are 1 mm each, whereas the detectors adjacent to the central rows are of increasing thickness, with

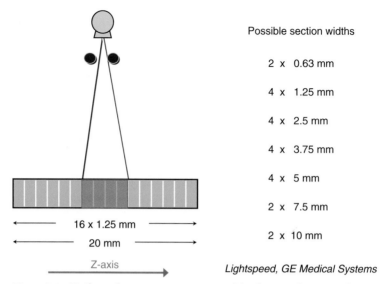

Possible section widths

2 x 0.63 mm

4 x 1.25 mm

4 x 2.5 mm

4 x 3.75 mm

4 x 5 mm

2 x 7.5 mm

2 x 10 mm

Lightspeed, GE Medical Systems

Figure 3.8. Uniform element arrays were one of the detector designs in the first-generation MDCT scanner. They consisted of individual detectors all of same dimensions. Also shown are the possible detector configurations that could be set for data acquisition. The product of individual detector thickness (T) and the number of detector elements (N) defines the total x-ray beam width (N*T) used during data acquisition.

the outermost detector row of 5 mm thick. By collimating half of the two innermost 1-mm wide detector arrays of 4 multiple-row detector scanners, a slice collimation of 2 × 0.5 mm could be obtained. By partially collimating the next arrays, 4 × 1-mm slices was obtained. By adding the innermost two detector rows yielded 4 × 2.5-mm collimation (Table 3.2)

One rationale behind this approach was to minimize absorption of x-rays by septa separating the detectors, which reduced the geometric efficiency. Siemens Medical Systems (Erlangen, Germany) and Philips Medical Systems (Eindhoven, the Netherlands) adopted this type of detector array designs in the four-slice MDCT scanners only. This type of detector array design is not used in later-generation MDCT scanners.

Hybrid Element Arrays. The third type of design incorporated features of uniform and nonuniform design (Fig. 3.10). This detector array is composed of thin detectors (0.5 mm) at center and thick detectors on either side of the central detectors. For example, in one of the

| Table 3.1 | Available detector configuration and available slice widths for image reconstruction on a four-slice MDCT scanner with uniform detector array design |

Detector configuration, N × T in mm	X-ray beam width, mm	Available slice widths for image reconstruction
2 × 0.625	1.25	0.63 and 1.25 mm
4 × 1.25	5	1.25 and 2.5 mm
4 × 2.5	10	2.5, 3.75, and 5.0 mm
4 × 3.75	15	3.75, 5.0, and 7.5 mm
4 × 5	20	5.0, 7.5, and 10.0 mm

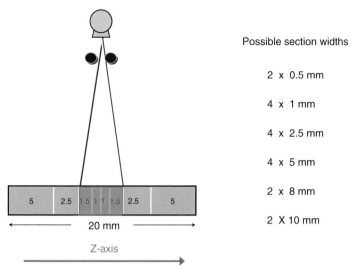

Possible section widths

2 x 0.5 mm

4 x 1 mm

4 x 2.5 mm

4 x 5 mm

2 x 8 mm

2 X 10 mm

Volume Zoom, Siemens Medical Systems

Figure 3.9. Nonuniform element arrays were one of the detector design in the first-generation MDCT scanner consisted of detectors with variable dimensions. In this design, the detector elements are smaller in dimension at the center and larger in dimension for the detectors away from the center. Shown also are the possible detector configurations that could be set for data acquisition.

four-slice MDCT scanners, there are four thin detectors of 0.5 mm at center and 15 detectors of 1 mm width on either side of the central detectors, for a total z-axis coverage of 32 mm per x-ray tube rotation around the gantry (Table 3.3). Toshiba Medical Systems (Nasu, Japan) introduced this type of detector array design.

For slice thickness larger than the minimum thickness of the detector array, the signals from several elements are combined in the z-direction, amplified, and converted to a digital signal. The aforementioned broad classification of detector-array design is helpful for discussing the next generation of MDCT scanners.

In MDCT, there is no postpatient collimation, as commonly found in the SDCT (except for the small septa or pieces of material that separate each detector in the x–y plane, which is slightly extended beyond the detector surface, not real septa). Instead, all collimation occurs at the x-ray tube end. Often, the detectors in z-direction use dividers between different detector rows that are opaque to the scintillation light produced during x-ray interactions in each detector elements (thus blocking cross-talk) but, at the same time, they are transparent to the incident x-ray radiation reaching detector in an oblique direction. This is critical especially for the peripheral detectors to

Table 3.2	Available detector configuration and available slice widths for image reconstruction on a four-slice MDCT scanner with nonuniform detector array design	
Detector configuration, N × T in mm	**X-ray beam width, mm**	**Available slice widths for image reconstruction**
2 × 0.5	1	0.5, 0.75, 1, 1.25, 1.5, and 2 mm
4 × 1.0	4	1, 1.25, 1.5, 2, 3, 4, 5, 6, 7, 8, and 10 mm
4 × 2.5	10	3, 4, 5, 6, 7, 8, and 10 mm
4 × 5	20	6, 7, 8, and 10 mm

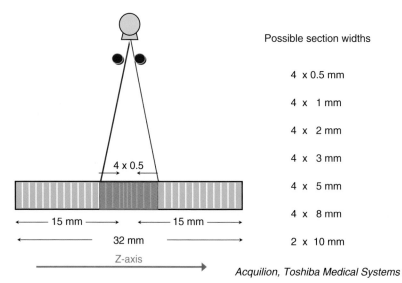

Possible section widths

4 x 0.5 mm

4 x   1 mm

4 x   2 mm

4 x   3 mm

4 x   5 mm

4 x   8 mm

2 x 10 mm

Acquilion, Toshiba Medical Systems

Figure 3.10. Hybrid element arrays were one of the detector design in the first-generation MDCT scanner reflected detector design of both uniform and variable thickness. Hence this design is appropriately named. In this design, the detector elements consisted of set of smaller thickness at the center and set of detector of larger dimensions on either side of the central detectors. Also shown are the possible detector configurations that could be set for data acquisition.

maintain dose efficiency. This effect increases dose efficiency but also makes the detector slightly more susceptible to scattered radiation reaching the detector. This highlights the capability to define the slice width by an electronic combination of signals, whereas the collimators close to the x-ray source determines the total x-ray beam width.

In MDCT the reconstructed slice thickness is always equal to or greater than the detector elements used in the CT scanner. One cannot reconstruct slices smaller than the dimension of the detector elements. For example, in a MDCT scanner with a detector width of 0.5 mm, one cannot reconstruct slices smaller than 0.5 mm; usually, the reconstructed slice thickness is greater than the defined detector width. The reasons for this widening are many-fold and are discussed in later chapters. The interpolation algorithms used in the reconstruction of the helical CT data are one of the factors in the widening of the reconstructed slice thickness.

Within 3 years of introducing first-generation MDCT scanners capable of yielding four slices

Table 3.3	Available detector configuration and available slice widths for image reconstruction on a four-slice MDCT scanner with hybrid detector array design	
Detector configuration, $N \times T$ in mm	**X-ray beam width (mm)**	**Available slice widths for image reconstruction**
4 × 0.5	2.0	0.5–2.0 mm in 0.5-mm increments
4 × 1	4	1–4 mm in 1-mm increments
4 × 2	8	2–10 mm in 1-mm increments
4 × 3	12	3–12 mm in 1-mm increments
4 × 4	16	4–16 mm in 1-mm increments
4 × 5	20	5–20 mm in 1-mm increments
4 × 8	32	8–32 mm in 1-mm increments

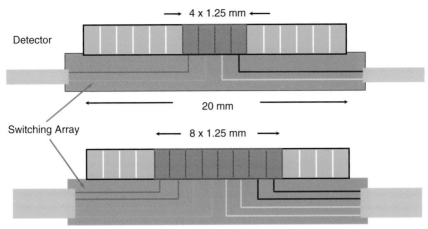

Figure 3.11. DAS channels: four versus eight. This figure illustrates the difference between MDCT scanners capable of yielding four and eight slices per gantry rotation. The main difference between the two systems is the availability of increased number of DAS channels.

per gantry rotation, vendors introduced MDCT scanners capable of yielding 8 and 16 slices. With eight-slice MDCT scanners, the detector array design still remained the same; however, the number of DAS channels was increased from four to eight, thereby allowing acquisition of eight simultaneous channels of data (Fig. 3.11).

The next major developmental stage in MDCT was the arrival of 16-slice MDCT scanners. A common aspect among all MDCT vendors was that all used a hybrid detector design in their scanners (Fig. 3.12). All scanners are limited to only 16 channels per rotation (Fig. 3.13). Because most of these scanners can complete half a second rotation per gantry, one could simultaneously obtain up to 32 slices in 1 second. The 16-slice MDCT scanners had remarkable improvement in terms of detector efficiency and, in addition, the scanning protocols became simplified over the previous generation of MDCT scanners (Figs. 3.14 and 3.15). Users could either scan in thin- or thick-slice acquisition mode. For example, one can scan 16 × 0.75 mm to yield a total of sixteen 0.75-mm slices, covering a scan volume of 12 mm (Fig. 3.16) or scan with 16 × 1.5 mm to yield sixteen 1.5-mm slices, covering 24 mm (Fig. 3.17).

Depending on the scan acquisition mode, users can then reconstruct into variety of slice thickness, but always equal to or greater than the acquired slice thickness (Fig. 3.18). Sixteen-slice MDCT scanners have the capability to image the most challenging organ in the human body—the heart. In fact, the challenge to perform cardiac imaging has become the driving forces behind further development in MDCT technology. Although MDCT scanners have helical-scan capability, axial or step and shoot acquisition also is possible. The step-and-shoot method of acquisition is often used during cardiac CT imaging, especially during calcium scoring (more details about cardiac imaging can be found in later chapter).

With regard to scan volume coverage, as shown in Figure 3.19 compared with SDCT, the MDCT scanners can cover large scan volume for similar scan time or scan same volume in shorter scan time (Table 3.4). In Figure 3.19, SDCT scanner required nearly 30 s to cover the scan volume of 150 mm. While keeping similar scan parameters, a four-slice MDCT scanner could cover up to 1000 mm in 30 s, whereas a 16-slice MDCT scanner took only 10 s to cover 1000 mm (Fig. 3.20). This is a remarkable advantage of scanning faster or covering larger scan volume, because scans that can be obtained within a single breath-hold present a clear advantage in cardiac imaging, pediatric imaging, and in trauma imaging.

The challenges in cardiac CT imaging and the need for greater spatial and temporal resolution led to the development of MDCT scanner with even greater slice capability. The next

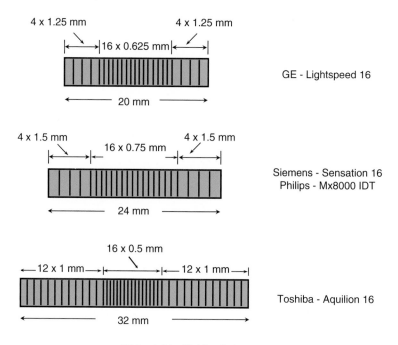

*Mahesh M, CliniCardio VascImg Textbook, pp 1-77, 2004

Figure 3.12. Detector designs used in the second-generation MDCT scanners capable of yielding 16 slices per gantry rotation. A common feature among these MDCT scanners is that all the detector designs are hybrid element arrays with thin detectors in the center and thick detectors on either side of the central detector elements. From Mahesh M, Clini Cardio Vasc Img Textbook, pp 1–77, 2004, with permission.)

MDCT scanners had the capability to yield 32 slices per gantry rotations. With a scan time less than 0.5 s, the manufacturers of these CT scanners claimed to yield 64 slices in 1 s (Fig. 3.21). The introduction of 64-slice MDCT scanners was the next major milestone in the MDCT series. In 64-slice MDCT scanners, all three major manufacturer (Toshiba, GE, and Philips) use uniform detector array design, whereas the fourth manufacturer (Siemens) uses the hybrid

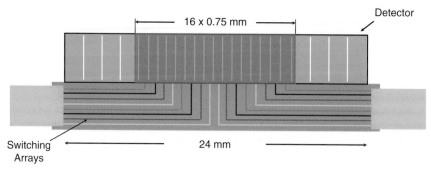

Figure 3.13. Demonstration of how detector elements are used in a 16-slice MDCT scanners. As shown, a 16-slice MDCT scanner consisted of 16 DAS channels to yield 16 slices per gantry rotation.

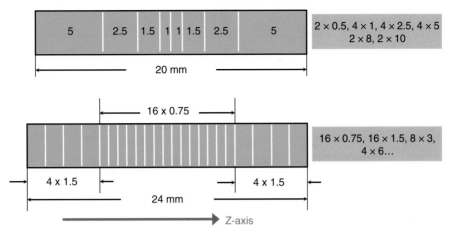

Siemens Medical Systems

Figure 3.14. Detector evolution: four versus 16 slices per rotation. Shown here is comparison of the detector elements between nonuniform elements array design (four-slice MDCT) and hybrid detector design (16-slice MDCT) and the possible detector configuration for data acquisition between the two detector designs.

detector array design (Fig. 3.22 and Table 3.5). If the number of detectors available are 16 or 64 and each of the detectors is only 1.25 mm or 0.625 mm in dimension, then the maximum coverage is 16 × 1.25 mm, equal to 20 mm, or 64 × 0.625 mm, equal to 40 mm. Although slices of variable thickness—1.25 or 2.5 mm or 5 mm—can be reconstructed, the maximum scan volume still cannot exceed the maximum x-ray beam coverage, for example, 20-mm or 40-mm as indicated in the aforementioned example.

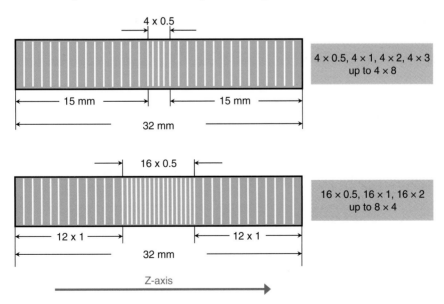

Toshiba Medical Systems

Figure 3.15. Detector evolution: four versus 16 slices per rotation. Shown here is comparison of the detector elements between the two hybrid detector designs (four-slice versus 16-slice MDCT) and the possible detector configuration for data acquisition between the two systems.

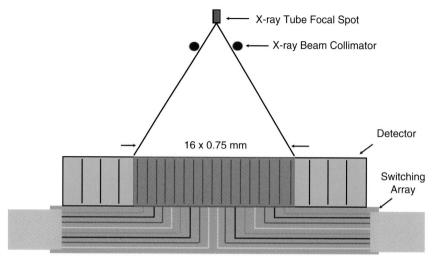

Figure 3.16. Illustration of detector configuration for 16 × 0.75 mm. Shown here is the detector configuration in which each of the 16 DAS channels collect data from 16 individual detector elements only. The total x-ray beam width is 12 mm (16 × 0.75 mm) and can be modified with different detector configuration. Data acquired in this way are used to reconstruct individual slices. The minimum slice thickness that can be obtained with this configuration is 0.75 mm or greater.

Image Reconstruction with MDCT

Before discussing the methods of image reconstruction with MDCT, it is important to recognize that reconstructing images from helical data is more complicated than in conventional CT reconstruction. In conventional CT, the images are reconstructed based on the principle of the filtered-back-projection method, where the attenuation measurements acquired around an object are projected onto the image place. One

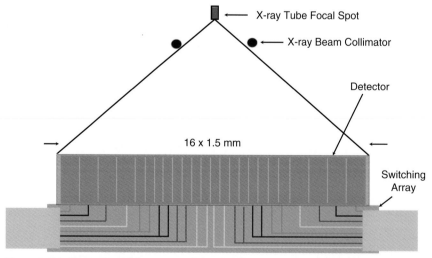

Figure 3.17. Illustration of detector configuration for 16 × 1.5 mm. Shown here is the detector configuration in which each of the 16 DAS channels collect data from 16 individual detector elements only. The total x-ray beam width is 24 mm (16 × 1.5 mm) and can be modified with different detector configuration. Data acquired in this way are used to reconstruct individual slices. The minimum slice thickness that can be obtained with this configuration is 1.5 mm or greater.

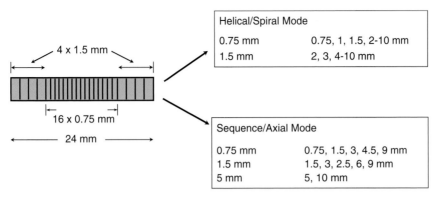

Figure 3.18. Illustrated here are the possible scan modes with respective acquisition and possible reconstructed slices obtained with a 16-slice MDCT scanner.

condition for this method is that all the data should be available on the same image plane. However, with helical CT acquisition using SDCT and MDCT, the acquisition data, except at a single location, do not lie on the same plane. Therefore, only after the development of interpolation algorithms did the image reconstruction of spiral/helical CT scan became feasible.

Among the various types of interpolation algorithms, the most common types are the linear interpolation algorithms (360 degrees + fan angle) and more advanced interpolation algorithms (180 degrees + fan angle). The linear interpolation algorithms are used to average the data from the same projection angle in front of and behind the image position (Fig. 3.23). Because the data used for reconstruction could extend from 360 degrees before to 360 degrees after the image place, the slices reconstructed

with this type of interpolation data could result in slices thicker (30–40% more) than the actual collimated width.

However, the more advanced interpolation algorithms exploit the fact that the data repeats in a 360 degree CT scanning, and each projection value is measured twice by two opposing rays. Therefore, by proper data sorting, it is possible to create a virtual second spiral data set (conjugated data) from which the interpolation can be done reducing the interpolation distance by half (Fig. 3.23). By doing so, the reconstructed slice thickness is more close to the actual collimated width; however, the images are slightly noisier because the image involves few data points along the longitudinal direction than the images obtained with 360-degree linear interpolation methods. The choice of the type of interpolation algorithms involves a trade-off between greater spatial

Table 3.4	Comparison of scan-time between SDCT and MDCT				
			Total scan time, seconds		
Scan region	**Distance, cm**	**Slice thickness, mm**	**SDCT**[a]	**MDCT**[b]
Head	20	8	16.7	2.1
Neck	15	5	20.0	2.5
Chest	30	8	25.0	3.1
Abdomen	20	8	16.7	2.1
Pelvis	20	8	16.7	2.1
Total scan time			95.1	11.9

[a]1-second scan, pitch 1.5.
[b]0.5-second scan, pitch equivalent to 1.5.

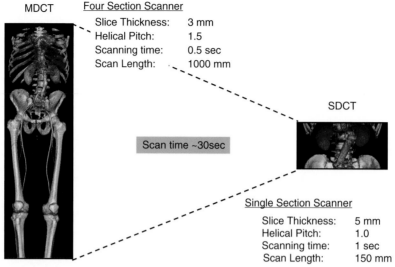

Figure 3.19. Illustrating the scan coverage possible with a four-slice MDCT scanner compared with a SDCT scanner for similar scan techniques and scan duration. A four-slice MDCT scanner has the potential to cover a 1000-mm scan length compared with 150-mm scan length with SDCT for a 30 second scan. (From Toshiba Medical Systems, Nasu, Japan, with permission).

resolution (thin slices and more noisy images with 180-degree advanced linear interpolation algorithms) and lesser image noise (thicker slices and less image noise as with 360-degree linear interpolation algorithms).

Reconstruction of MDCT data involves an even more complex method to interpolate data between not only a single helical data and its conjugate data set but also the data streams from multiple detector sets. Similar to SDCT, the data

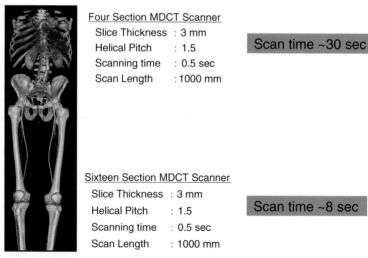

Figure 3.20. Illustrating the scan coverage possible with a 16-slice MDCT scanner compared with a four-slice MDCT scanner for similar scan techniques. A 16-slice MDCT scanner has the potential to cover 1000 mm scan length in less than 10 seconds compared with the scan duration of nearly 30 seconds with a four-slice scanner. (FromToshiba Medical Systems, Nasu, Japan, with permission).

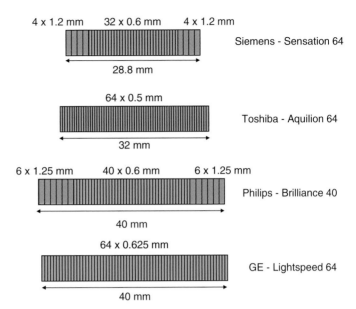

Figure 3.21. Detector elements array design for MDCT scanners with capability to yield more than 32 slices per gantry rotation.

in MDCT are interpolated either by 360-degree interpolations or 180-degree interpolations. In addition, unique with MDCT data is the use of the z-filter interpolation method. Z-filter interpolation uses not only the two projections from the detectors that are closest to the scan plane but also adjacent projections. These projections are weighed according to their distance from the scan plane. The z-filter controls the slice width

of the slice profile of the reconstructed images (Fig. 3.24), which will allow the user to select the size and shape of the filter for more control over the effective slice thickness versus noise trade-offs. There are many variations in the type of z-filtering methods developed by different manufacturers, thus providing variations in the availability of the selections for the reconstructed slice thickness. With the z-filtering method, it is

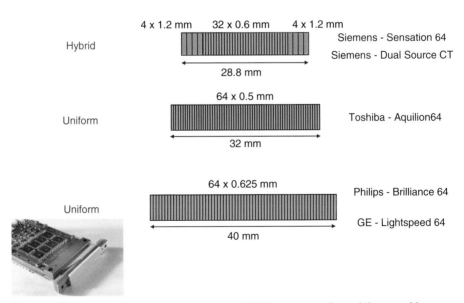

Figure 3.22. Detector elements array design for MDCT scanners with capability to yield 64 slices per gantry rotation. Two distinct types of detector designs, uniform and hybrid detector designs, are used in the 64-slice MDCT scanners.

Table 3.5	Available detector configuration and total x-ray beam width in 16- and 64-slice MDCT scanners	

Detector configuration, $N \times T$ in mm	X-ray beam width, mm
16×0.625	10
16×1.25	20
16×0.75	12
16×1.5	24
16×0.5	8
16×1.0	16
16×2	32
64×0.625	40
32×0.6^{a}	19.2
24×1.2^{a}	28.8
64×0.5	32

[a] Yields 64 slices per gantry rotation with Straton x-ray tube that has two fluctuating focal spots and each detector is double sampled? (more discussion can be found in later chapters).

key to understand that the reconstructed slice thickness can only be greater and not smaller than the DAS channel widths for the type of data acquisition with MDCT scanning (for example, 4 $\times$ 1.25 mm can yield a slice thickness of 1.25 mm or greater and not less than 1.25 mm).

With increasing number of detectors (16 and higher), the complexity of image reconstruction with MDCT increases as the result of increasing cone beam of the projected x-rays in the longitudinal direction. Many different approaches have

been taken to develop cone beam reconstruction methods to accommodate increasing cone-angle of the x-ray beam in longitudinal direction. The details of such methods can be found among the list of suggested reading materials.

Dual-Source CT and 320-Row MDCT. The demand for greater temporal and spatial resolution further led to the development of the dual-source CT (DSCT) scanner (Siemens) and 320-row MDCT scanner (Toshiba). In DSCT, there are two x-ray tubes positioned at 90 degrees apart with two sets of detectors, each capable of yielding 64 slices per gantry rotation. The major advantage of this scanner is the improved temporal resolution (Fig. 3.25). The scan field of view is smaller when both the x-ray tubes are used for scanning compared with scanning with single x-ray tube. The scanner is designed predominantly to perform cardiac imaging. Details on DSCT are discussed in later chapters.

Similarly, the demand for greater spatial resolution first led to the development of prototype 256-row MDCT scanner (Toshiba), which can cover the entire heart in one gantry rotation (256×0.5 mm = 12.8 cm beam width at iso-center). In this type of scanner, it is possible to obtain complete data from one heart cycle and has the potential to reduce radiation dose and motion artifacts. In 2007, this vendor (Toshiba) introduced 320-row MDCT scanner with 16 cm coverage at iso-center per gantry rotation.

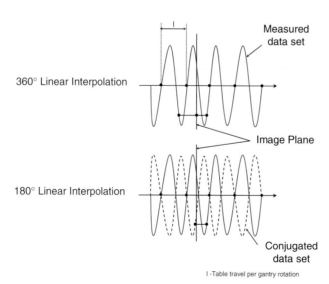

Figure 3.23. Types of interpolation methods used for spiral CT data. A 360-degree interpolation algorithm interpolates from 360 degrees behind and 360 degrees in front of the desired image plane, whereas the 180-degree linear interpolation method interpolates only 180 degrees of data behind and in front of the desired image plane tending minimal spread of the reconstructed slice thickness.

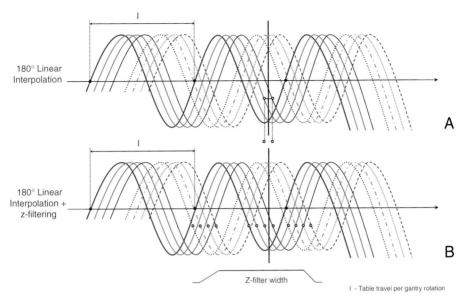

Figure 3.24. Illustration of the type of interpolation method used in MDCT scanners. Shown here are the two types of interpolation method. **A:** 180-degree linear interpolation method interpolates between the 180-degree linear interpolation method interpolates data from adjacent detector data. **B:** 180-degree linear interpolation with z-filtering method. Z-filtering method allows variation of effective slice thickness.

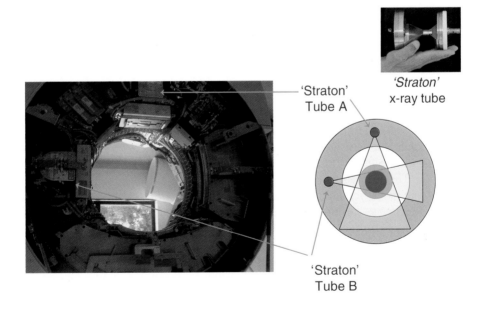

Figure 3.25. Shown is the DSCT gantry with two x-ray tubes "*Straton*" along with two detector systems. Also illustrated here is the dimension of scan field of view available for each x-ray tube and detector combination. The detector system aligned with tube A is the larger of the two detector systems and is similar to SDCT system. The second detector system aligned with tube B is smaller of the two yielding smaller field of view.

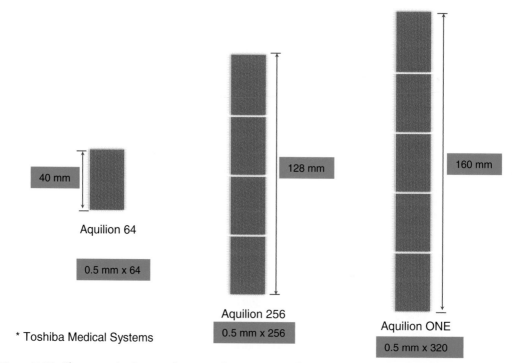

Figure 3.26. Shown are the detector element and scan coverage for 256- and 320-row MDCT scanner compared with 64-row MDCT scanner from the same manufacturer. (From Toshiba Medical Systems, Nasu, Japan, with permission). The maximum scan coverage with 320-row MDCT scanner is 160 mm at the scanner isocenter with the motivation to cover the entire heart in a single gantry rotation.

Details on 256 and 320-row MDCT are discussed in later chapters.

Advantages of MDCT. The advantages of multiple-row detector technology can be broadly divided into three categories. (a) The ability to obtain a large number of thin slices resulting in greater spatial resolution in both axial and longitudinal direction. This is important in terms of obtaining isotropic spatial resolution, i.e., cubic voxels, wherein the images are equally sharp in any plane traversing the scanned volume. This capability is reasonably obtained with multiple sections of sub-millimeter thickness. Ideally the true three-dimensional radiograph would have cubic voxels of <1 mm in size, over large volumes, acquired with very short times within a reasonable breath-hold. (b) The speed can be used for fast imaging of large volume of tissue with variable slice thickness. This is particularly useful in cardiac imaging studies, and studies where patient motion is a limiting factor such as in trauma or pediatric cases. With a 4-slice

system and a 0.5-section rotation, the volume data can be acquired eight times faster than with the single slice, 1-s scanner. With 16- and 64-slice systems and rotation times of less than 0.5 s, the volume data are acquired at an even greater rate than that of first-generation MDCT scanners. With 256- and 320-row MDCT, the coverage of entire heart in a single gantry rotation at scan time less than 0.5 s is a reality that leads to acquiring cardiac data in a single heartbeat. (c) The other main advantage of MDCT is the ability to cover large volumes in short scanning times. The volume coverage and speed performance in MDCT scanners is better than its counterpart SDCT without compromising image quality. The fast rotation times and large volume coverage provides improved multiplanar reconstruction and three-dimensional images with reduced image artifacts and have led to a lot of new clinical applications.

One of the consequences of MDCT scanning is the radiation exposure. The radiation exposures in MDCT protocol are not insignificant and therefore need special attention when designing new clinical protocols. More on radiation dose and strategies to reduce dose are discussed in details in later chapters. The discussion on MDCT scanners is never complete because it has been a moving target the past few years. Every year newer scanners with greater number of slices are introduced to the marketplace. The so-called "slice wars" keep raging and with 320-row scanners, the slice wars be reaching a plateau. The challenges of cardiac imaging and functioning imaging fuel the development of CT technology to perform with greater spatial and temporal resolution.

4

Major Components of MDCT Scanners

In this chapter, we will discuss the major components of a computed tomography (CT) scanner. The two major components of a CT scanner are the CT gantry and the patient table. For most CT units, they are similar in design and occupy similar floor space (Fig. 4.1). The multiple detector design and configurations were discussed in detail in Chapter 3, and the components, such as the gantry, x-ray tube, collimators, filters, and the patient table are described here. In addition to these components, there are other essential components, such as power generators, electronics, computers and controls, and air conditioning. The main components inside the CT gantry are as shown in Figure 4.2.

CT Gantry and Slip-Ring Technology

The mechanical design in CT is an engineering challenge. The components of a CT gantry (Fig. 4.3) represents a mass typically ranging from 3300 lbs (1500 kg) to more than 4400 lbs (2000 kg) that has the potential to generate massive centrifugal force (2–30 g) of gravity. This poses even greater demand on the technological design of CT gantry to attain fast gantry rotation speed with such a huge mass and yet sustain very high centrifugal forces created as the result of the high speed.

All MDCT scanners consist of a slip-ring technology, which allows for continuous rotation of x-ray tube and detector elements around patients without having to stop scanning to

unwind the wire connecting the various components (which is a limitation of conventional and nonhelical CT scanners). Slip rings are electromechanical devices consisting of circular electrical conductive rings and brushes that transmit electrical energy across a moving interface. All power and control signals from the stationary parts of the scanner system are communicated to the rotating frame through the slip ring (Fig. 4.4). The slip-ring design consists of sets of parallel conductive rings concentric to the gantry axis that connect to the tube, detectors, and control circuits by sliding contractors. These *sliding contractors* allow the scan frame to rotate continuously with no need to stop between rotations to rewind system cables (Fig. 4.4). This engineering advancement resulted initially from a desire to reduce interscan delay and improve throughput. The slip-ring gantry allows data from MDCT detectors to transfer optically or by high-frequency brushes touching the outer rings.

Typically, most MDCT scanners have a gantry with an opening of up to 70 cm in diameter. Although the CT gantry has a physical aperture of approximately 70 cm in diameter, the actual sampling area where the attenuation measurements are made is smaller than the physical opening and the actual sampling area usually is 50–55 cm in diameter (Fig. 4.5). Because the sampling area is smaller than the physical gantry opening, the CT image can be degraded, resulting in failure to image an appropriate part of the patient's shoulder or hip that lies outside the sampling area. The plane of the gantry opening is called the *axial plane* (in-plane or x–y plane) and

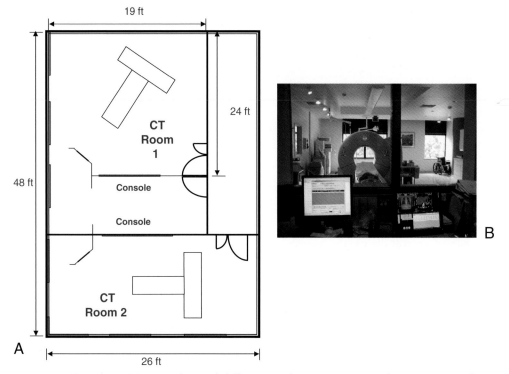

Figure 4.1. Typical MDCT scanner layout: (**A**) illustration showing CT suites with common control area; (**B**) photograph of the examination room.

the longitudinal direction that is in and out of the gantry is noted as *z-direction*. Certain specially designed CT gantries for radiation oncology (i.e., the open-bore gantry) or in hybrid scanners (such as positron emission tomography [PET]/ CT scanners, the CT gantry aperture is large to match PET gantry) have openings up to 90 cm. In addition, certain manufacturers even provide options to reconstruct image area of up to the gantry opening (virtual image reconstruction).

CT X-Ray Tube

The x-ray tube is the most important component for the success of any x-ray examination. CT is one of the most demanding x-ray tube applications. Compared with any other diagnostic x-ray application, CT x-ray tubes are subjected to far greater thermal loads. In a way, progress in CT has been linked to the progress in CT x-ray tube technology. In early CT scanners, such as in first- and second-generation ones, stationary anode x-ray tubes were used because the long scan times meant

the instantaneous power level was low and long scan times also allowed for heat dissipation. However, the introduction of spiral scanning with MDCT's precursor, SDCT, placed new demands on x-ray tubes, and progress in MDCT became possible only because of the further development of high-power x-ray tubes with greater heat dissipation capability.

Demand for greater temporal resolution implies shorter scan time and requires a high-power x-ray tube that can deliver larger x-ray photons in shortest time achievable. This demand led to several technical advances in component design to achieve the high power levels and address the problems of target temperature, heat storage, and dissipation. For example, the tube envelope, cathode assembly, and anode assemblies (including anode rotation and target design) have been redesigned. Heat storage capacities varied from 1 to 3 million heat units (MHUs) in early third-generation CT scanners. As scan times have decreased, anode heat capacities have increased by as much as a factor of three, preventing the need for cooling

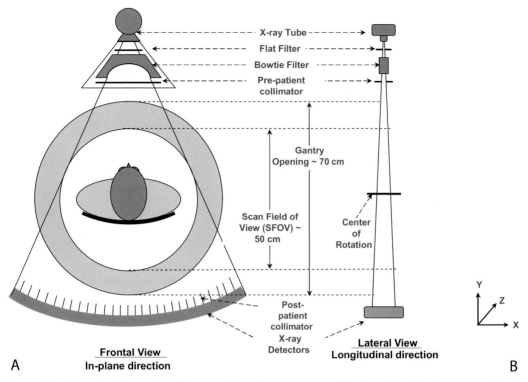

Figure 4.2. Schematic diagram of a CT gantry with major components: **(A)** frontal view (in-plane or x–y plane) and **(B)** lateral view (longitudinal plane or y–z plane)

delays during most clinical procedures, and tubes with capacities of 5–9 MHU are available. In addition, improvement in heat dissipation rate (KHU/min) has increased the heat storage capacity on modern x-ray tubes by using oil cooled rotating anodes with efficient thermal dissipation and other design features.

The working life of tubes used to date ranges from 10,000 to 40,000 hours, compared with 1000 hours, which is typical of conventional CT

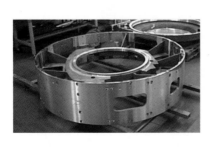
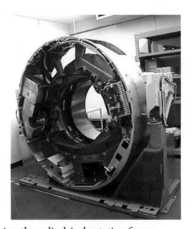

Figure 4.3. Photograph of a CT gantry showing the cylindrical rotation frame designed to withstand 5–20 *g* force created during gantry rotation times of less than 500 ms. (From Toshiba Medical Systems, with permission.)

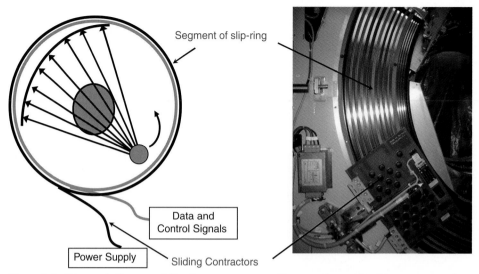

Figure 4.4. Schematic diagram of slip-ring gantry system. Photograph on right shows segment of slip-ring gantry with sliding contractors powering the gantry and transmitting the data and control signals.

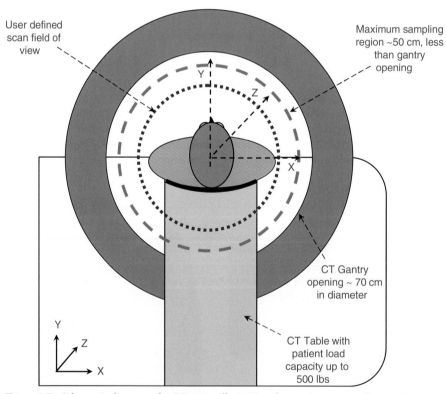

Figure 4.5. Schematic diagram of a CT gantry illustrating the maximum sampling region (~50 cm in diameter). The user-defined scan field of view is within the maximum sampling region. Also illustrated is the x–y plane defined as the in-plane or axial plane and the z-axis indicating the longitudinal direction.

tubes. They are now specified by the number of slices an x-ray tube can scan without having to stop for x-ray tube cooling. Tube life that can scan for more than half-a-million slices or greater are not uncommon now. Increased tube life translates to a reduced operational cost and reduced scanner downtime. Also key to any smooth clinical operation is the length of the downtime between repairs. A shorter/quicker x-ray tube replacement process is imperative because it means less interruption to the daily clinical operation.

Because many of the engineering changes increase the mass of the tube, much of the design effort also was dedicated to reduce the mass to better withstand increasing gantry rotational rates required by ever faster scan times. Typical values for x-ray tube maximum power ranges from 20 kW to 150 kW, with high voltage ranging from 80 kV to 140 kV and tube current ranging as high as 800 mA. The maximum power ratings are the limit that cannot be sustained over a longer period of time.

Each MDCT manufacturer has improved or developed better-designed x-ray tubes to meet the demand of scanning thinner slices and covering larger anatomy yet delivering the required amount of x-ray flux. In fact, the x-ray tubes are more efficiently used in MDCT compared with SDCT scanners because the x-ray beam is wider (beam width = N × T, for example, with

MDCT, 64 × 0.625 mm = 40 mm) allowing greater x-ray flux produced by the x-ray tube in creating a CT image compared to SDCT (Beam width = T, for example with SDCT, T = 1 mm).

Although the x-ray production is inefficient (1% x-ray production versus 99% heat production), greater emphasis has been attempted to achieve faster heat and also to produce more efficient and quality x-rays by absorbing off-focal radiation. For example, the large heat capacities are achieved with thick graphite backing of target disks, anode diameters of 200 mm or more, improved high temperature rotor bearings and metal housings with ceramic insulators (Fig. 4.6) among other factors.

One MDCT manufacturer introduced total redesigned x-ray tube similar to electron-beam CT technology, where both the cathode and anode enclosed in a vacuum container rotate inside an enclosure cooled by oil. The *Straton* tube has an anode of approximately 120 mm in diameter, which is much smaller than other high-power x-ray tubes and allows a greater reduction in mass and size (Fig. 4.7). The Straton tube works similarly to electron-beam CT technology, where an external magnetic field modulates the electron beam exiting the cathode within the tube and allows overlapping sampling of x-rays. Because of this method, although the CT scanner has only "X" number of distinct detectors (e.g., 32 of each 0.6 mm size), it can allow "2X" the number

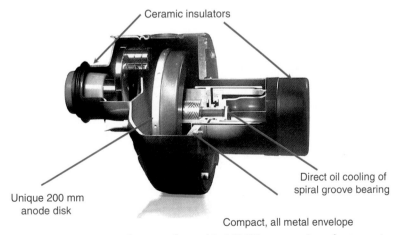

Figure 4.6. Rotating anode x-ray tube used in MDCT scanners. Large heat capacities (5–8 MHU) are achieved with large anode disks and custom designed metal housing with ceramic insulators. (From Philips Medical Systems, Shelton, CT, with permission).

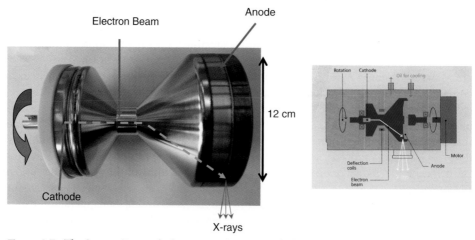

Figure 4.7. The Straton X-ray tube has unique features, including an electron beam focused by an external magnetic field that modulates the beam to strike the directly cooled anode tube, creating "flying" focal spots in both in-plane and longitudinal direction. The entire cathode and anode assembly rotates and the anode is cooled externally by circulating oil in the tube housing allowing efficient heat dissipation. (From Siemens Medical Systems, with permission.)

of slices ($2 \times 32 \times 0.6$ or 64 slices of 0.6 mm size) because of double sampling.

Another aspect of x-ray tube design apart from heat dissipation is the challenge to minimize off-focal radiation. Off-focal radiation is caused when secondary electrons bounce off the x-ray tube anode and are directed towards the patient and detectors. If such x-rays are not diminished, the net effect from off-focal radiation is to increase radiation exposure and deteriorate contrast resolution. MDCT manufacturers have redesigned the x-ray tube to include a specially designed grounded aperture or backscattered electron suppression ring to absorb recoil electrons with the intention of reducing off-focal radiation. Manufacturers also have adopted designs in which the anode is on a shaft that makes it more stable during faster rotations and allows it to reduce the distance between the cathode and anode, making it more efficient in terms of heat dissipation and has large heat capacity (7.5 MHU) (Fig. 4.8). Overall, because the x-ray tube is a key component of a CT scanner, major innovations in x-ray tube design and enhancements in heat dissipation

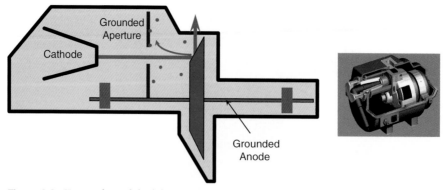

Figure 4.8. X-ray tube with high heat capacity (7.5 MHU) has unique features such as grounded aperture to absorb recoil electrons and to reduce off-focal x-rays. In addition, grounded anode provides stability for faster anode rotation and with large anode diameter yields efficient heat dissipation (from Toshiba Medical Systems, with permission).

and many other improvements have propelled the development of MDCT scanner technology.

CT Collimation

Collimation in CT may vary among scanner types but, in principle, they all offer the same functions, such as capability to reduce unnecessary radiation dose to patient and to define the x-ray beam edge for the CT scans. There are two types of collimators associated with CT scanners. First, the prepatient collimators, positioned close to x-ray tube, and second the postpatient collimators, positioned closer to the CT detectors (Fig. 4.9). The prepatient collimators reduces the x-ray beam roughly to the maximum beam anticipated for a given detector and geometry. The collimator blades are made up of lead materials and in the axial plane (in-plane or x–y plane) the blades are fixed by the fan angle required by the CT geometry to cover all the detector elements. However, in the longitudinal direction, the pre-patient collimators are varied to adjust the x-ray beam size.

For a nonhelical or in the SDCT scanners, the prepatient collimators not only reduce dose to the patient but also define the slice thickness of the imaging plane. However, in the MDCT

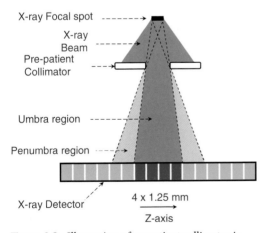

Figure 4.9. Illustration of prepatient collimator in MDCT scanners showing the umbra and penumbra region of the x-ray beam. In MDCT, there are no postpatient collimators in longitudinal direction; instead, postpatient collimation is generally performed electronically by the detector array, which also defines the slice thickness.

scanners the detector aperture defines the slice thickness and not the prepatient collimators. In MDCT scanners, the prepatient collimators define the total x-ray beam size and are based on the detector configurations (for example 16 × 0.75 mm = 12 mm corresponding to N × T, where N is the number of DAS channels and T is the width of each DAS channel).

In MDCT scanners, generally there are no postpatient collimators in the longitudinal direction. The postcollimation is conducted electronically and conforms to the size of the detector channel rather than any type of physical collimators. In fact, to ensure all detector cells receive equal amount of x-ray photons, the total x-ray beam width is set slightly larger than the detector size (N×T). In fact, in early MDCT scanners (four-slice systems), this condition led to the beam size being larger than the detector configuration and led to poor geometric efficiency in the longitudinal direction (discussion on geometric efficiency in MDCT scanners can be found in later chapters). The only types of collimation that are available on the postpatient side are in the in-plane or axial direction (Fig. 4.10) and are in the form of septa extending out of the detector cells all focused towards the focal spot of the x-ray tube.

CT Filters

There are different types of filters that are inserted in the x-ray portal on the side of the x-ray source in the CT scanner (Fig. 4.2). The common filter is the *flat shaped filter*, comprising aluminum or copper material, which absorbs most of the low-energy x-rays. In addition to the inherent filtration provided by the x-ray tube, flat filters absorb low energy x-rays and shift the resultant x-ray spectrum to higher energies (Fig. 4.11). The goal of shaping the spectrum of the x-ray beam by using physical absorbing filters in CT is to eliminate those low-energy photons that contribute to patient exposure but do not reach the detectors and therefore do not add to image information and image quality.

Bowtie Filters. In addition to flat filters, beam-shaping filters are introduced to provide

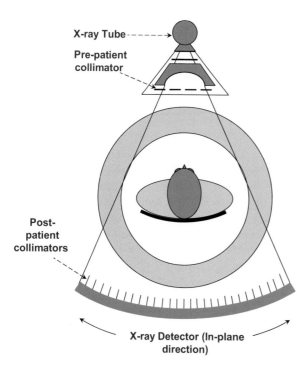

Figure 4.10. Illustration of postpatient collimators in the in-plane or axial direction in a MDCT scanner. The septa, made up of strong x-ray absorbing materials such as lead, extends out of the detector cells and is focused toward the x-ray focal spot with the intention of blocking scatter radiation from reaching the x-ray detectors.

an effective means to improve dose utilization. These so-called *bowtie filters* hardly absorb x-rays at the center but absorb off-axis rays to maintain a more uniform x-ray field at the detector, regardless of the position of the beam through the patient (Fig. 4.12). The bowtie filter allows reducing the surface dose to the patient without substantially increasing the noise in the image and it also helps in reducing x-ray scattering effects, thereby improving the signal-to-noise ratio in the image. The ideal bowtie filter is one that's tailored to the specific patient size and shape. Typically only a small set of bowtie filters (i.e., head and body) are available on CT systems. However, some CT manufacturers provide bowtie filters based on size of the scanning objects, such as small, medium, and large.

Choosing an inappropriate scan field of view can introduce wrong bowtie filter and therefore yield greater radiation dose and also incorrect image reconstruction. Others have introduced bowtie filters specifically designed for cardiac CT scan protocols that allow substantial dose reduction without increasing noise or otherwise affecting image quality in the reconstructed field

of view typically used in cardiac applications. Proper selection of bowtie filters based on patient size and imaging needs may result in dose savings of up to 50%.

CT Detectors

An equally important component of the entire CT system is the detectors. Like x-rays, CT detectors have experienced tremendous growth during the past 30 years. The MDCT designs are the latest in the detector design path. The main purpose is to convert x-ray energies exiting the patient into electrical signal used in the image formation. In CT detectors, the path of converting x-rays into electrical signal is achieved either by ionization chambers (mostly filled with Xenon gas under high pressure) or by solid-state detectors made up of scintillation materials that convert x-rays to light signals, which in turn are converted into electrical signals.

Across the various MDCT systems, all of the MDCT detector systems are made up of solid-state detectors. Although detail information regarding the structure, composition, and other details are not readily available and are mostly

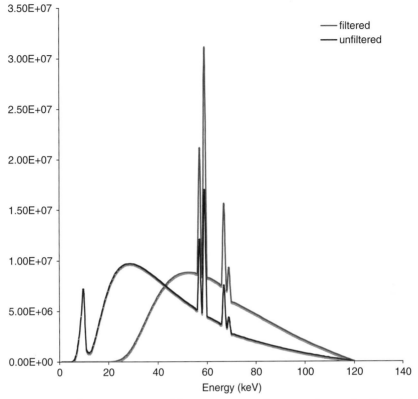

Figure 4.11. The average energy of the x-ray spectrum increases after passing through filter materials. Filter of variable thickness are introduced to harden the x-ray beam by removing low energy x-rays that do not contribute to CT image but increases patient surface dose.

proprietary, suffice to say that all MDCT systems are made up of solid-state detectors and have some sort of scintillation material that converts x-rays into light photons, which in turn converts them into electrical signal. Details about the configuration and how the detectors are used to derive at multiple slices per gantry rotation were discussed at length in Chapter 3.

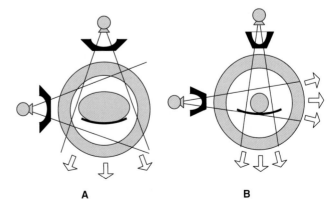

Figure 4.12. Bowtie filter is selected based on the anatomical size during a CT scan. **A:** Large bowtie filter for large anatomy. **B:** Small bowtie filter for small anatomy.

A

B

Table 4.1   Comparison chart of various key components for 64-slice MDCT scanners

MDCT manufacturer	GE	Philips	Siemens	Toshiba
MDCT model	LightSpeed VCT Select	Brilliance 64-Channel	Sensation 64	Aquilion 64 CFX
Components				
CT gantry opening, cm	70	70	70	72
Maximum SFOV, cm	50	50	50	50
CT X-ray tube				
Heat capacity, MHCI	8	8	0 Equivalent to 30 MHCI[a]	7.5
Power output, kW	100	60	80	72
Tube voltage, kVp	80, 100, 120, 140	80, 120, 140	80, 100, 120, 140	80, 100, 120, 135
Tube current, mA range	10–800	20–500	28–665	10–600
X-ray beam fan angle, degrees	56	57	54.4	49.2
CT detector	Hilight Ceramic matrix	Solid State GOS[b]	Ultra Fast Ceramic[b]	Solid State[b]
No. of detectors rows (longitudinal or in z-direction)	64	64	40	64
Smallest detector width, mm	0.625	0.625	0.6	0.5
No. of detector elements per row (in-plane or axial direction)	912	672	672	896
CT table max capacity, lbs	500	450	450	450

[a] Station tube.
[b] Patented, details not available.
SFOV, scan field of view.

CT Table

Apart from CT gantry and all its components, the next key component is the CT table or patient bed. The design of a CT table is also an ongoing challenge to the manufacturers. With obesity on the rise globally, increasing demand for tables that can accommodate greater weight poses greater design challenges. The two critical functions for a CT table are that the table should rise up and down (ranges from 30 to 100 cm) with precision and move at constant or variable speed in and out of the gantry (ranges up to 200 cm) with high precision. The movement of CT table especially in and out of the CT gantry is specified to a certain precision for up to certain weights. The influx of hybrid scanners (PET-CT) put even greater demand for precise bed movement because it can jeopardize quantification of pathology in CT. Most MDCT tables can accommodate patient weights up to 450 lbs and provide a precision of 1 to 2 mm, and specially designed CT tables can accommodate patient weights up to 600 lbs. Most CT tables are made up of carbon fiber materials that have least x-ray absorption capability.

Summary

There are number of components that comprise a MDCT scanner. The most important components, such as CT gantry, x-ray tube, collimators, filtration, and detection system, that are unique to MDCT scanners are listed in Table 4.1. Additional details about each of the components and also about the components that are not discussed in this chapter can be found among the list of suggested readings.

5

Scan Parameters and Image Quality in MDCT

In this chapter, we will discuss important parameters in computed tomography (CT) imaging that the CT operator controls and adjusts. We will then examine how various parameters influence the image quality and the radiation dose. Every CT user is comfortable with a particular set of techniques; therefore, techniques can be customized only if the CT user understands the role of each scan parameters and the trade-offs involved. For each scan parameter various steps that can be applied to lower the radiation dose without compromising image quality are discussed.

Scan Modes

Once the patient is brought into a CT suite, the CT technologist or user positions the patient on the CT table such that he or she is at the isocenter of the CT gantry to obtain optimal image quality and radiation dose. Before proceeding with axial CT scan series, the user first performs a *scout scan* or a *topograph scan*. This step enables the user to select the region for the axial CT scans. Scout scans also are known as the *topograph survey scan*, which are simply radiographs of the select region obtained with a low-scan technique yielding low radiation dose to patient. The x-ray tube is held stationary inside the CT gantry, and the table is translated through the CT gantry, resulting in a scout scan. Typically, the tube is positioned at zero degrees (top of the patient) within the CT gantry. The radiation dose to the patient is close to a typical radiographic exposure and accounts for a small percentage of total dose from

complete CT examination. As shown in Figure 5.1, the scout image allows user to select or mark the region for the axial series of scans. With dose-modulation techniques available (discussed later in Chapter 8), certain multidetector row CT (MDCT) scanners require two scout scans to apply dose-modulation techniques and are obtained in anteroposterior (AP) and lateral projection. In such situations, scout scans are used to estimate patient thickness in both AP and lateral projection, which are then used to vary the tube current during axial scans. Radiation dose from scout scan can be further reduced, not only by setting the scan techniques as low as possible but, in addition, if the x-ray tube is stationed underneath the patient (at 180 degrees) instead of on top of the patient (as done traditionally), additional reduction in the radiation dose also is possible. The following axial scan modes are available on MDCT scanners.

First, a *sequential scan mode*, an active scanning mode, is performed; second, a *helical* or series of spiral scanning; third, a *quick scan*; and fourth, a *dynamic* scan. Sequential scanning is similar to the conventional CT scanning wherein after each scan the table is moved to the next position before imaging the next region. This mode is also called as *step-and-shoot* scanning mode (Fig. 5.2A). These are incremental scans with slice-by-slice imaging capability in which there is no table movement during data acquisition. There is a minimum interscan delay between each slice as the table is moved to the next location. After the introduction of helical scanning mode, most CT scans protocols are

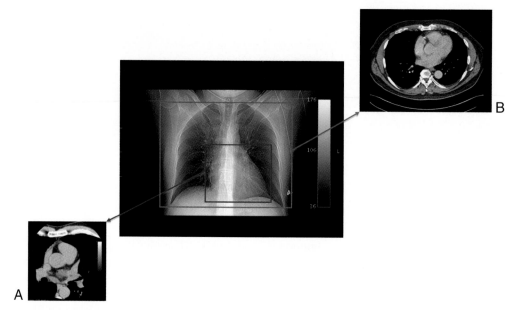

Figure 5.1. The scout scan image allow users to select or mark regions for the axial series of scans. Shown here are two cases: **(A)** a chest image based on the larger region selection and **(B)** a cardiac CT image confined to the smaller region marked on the scout scan.

performed helically. However, there are certain scans still performed in sequential scan mode. Among them are certain cranial CT scans and cardiac CT scans. Among the cardiac CT imaging, calcium scoring scans are predominantly performed in sequential scan mode. These days, with the aim of lowering radiation dose in CT angiography scans, sequential scan modes are adopted with prospective ECG triggering methods (for details, refer to Chapter 7). With large area detectors, such as 256- or 320-row detectors capable of scanning large anatomical area in a single sweep of the x-ray tube in the CT gantry, it appears that sequential scan mode may become the chosen scan mode of the future.

The second scan mode is *helical scan* mode, in which a continuous volume data acquisition is possible during which the data acquisition is synchronized with the table movement (Fig. 5.2B). The data acquisition and table movements are acquired simultaneously for the entire scan duration, which eliminates the interscan delay between the scan. The introduction of helical scan mode in 1980s was the evolutionary leap in the CT technology and, in fact, the advantages of helical scanning mode for three-dimensional

volume data acquisition were the impetus to the development of MDCT scanners.

Apart from these types of axial scans, there are other type of axial scan modes, such as the *quick scan* and *partial scan*. Often, the user who wants to verify location of the region of interest performs a quick full (360-degree) rotation scan. This scan can be performed at a low dose because the image is not used for any interpretation, only for ensuring positioning. A quick scan also used as a target scan can be performed in partial rotation of the x-ray tube (less than full rotation) and is known as a partial scan (Fig. 5.2C).

The fourth type of scan mode is *dynamic multiscan*. In dynamic multiscan, multiple continuous rotation of the x-ray tube is performed with the table position held constant (Fig. 5.2D). This particular type of scans are used for test bolus runs to estimate the time required for the contrast to reach the area of interest. During test bolus, the table is stationary and repeat scans are done until the contrast reaches the area of interest. The scanner then estimates the time before actual scans begins. These types of dynamic scans are also done during CT perfusion or CT fluoroscopy scans.

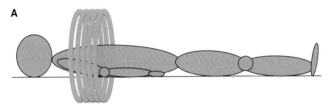

Sequential or 'Step and Shoot' scan mode

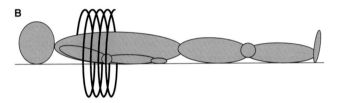

Helical or spiral scan mode

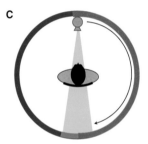

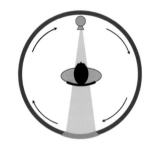

| Partial scan mode – Half-scan plus fan angle | Dynamic scan mode – Multiple continuous rotation of x-ray tube at same table position |

Figure 5.2. Type of axial scans. **A:** sequential or step-and-shoot scan mode performed in non-helical CT scanners. They also are performed in MDCT scanners, especially during cardiac CT scans in prospective scan mode with the goal of lowering radiation dose. **B:** Helical scan mode allows continuous data acquisition with patient movement synchronized with data acquisition. **C:** Partial scan mode performed with minimal rotation of the x-ray tube needed to create an image. **D:** dynamic multiscan mode involves multiple scans of the same region achieved by keeping the CT table in the same position.

Primary Scan Factors

Tube Voltage. Tube voltage is the potential difference maintained between the anode and cathode in an x-ray tube. It provides the energy to the electrons ejected by the x-ray filament to accelerate towards the anode. When electrons accelerating as the result of the potential difference initiated by the kilo-voltage peak (kVp) hit the anode, *Bremsstrahlung x-rays* are produced (for more details on the x-ray production, refer to basic medical physics textbooks listed under suggested reading materials). The tube voltage influences the nature of the x-rays produced.

Characteristics of *Bremsstrahlung x-rays* are that the x-rays of all different energies are produced. The average energy of x-rays coming out of the x-ray tube is usually one-third of the peak tube voltage (kVp).

Not all x-rays are suitable for imaging. Low-energy x-rays are absorbed on the skin surface and do not contribute to the image formation but increase the radiation dose to the patient. Therefore, like in any other radiographic procedure, the soft x-rays are absorbed by introducing beam filters in the path of the x-rays exiting out of the x-ray tube anode. With beam filters in the path of the x-rays, the exiting x-rays are hardened, and the overall energy of the x-rays is increased. This process. known as *beam hardening*, implies removal of soft x-rays from the exiting x-ray beam so that the remaining x-rays have higher average energies. For example, in Figure 5.3, the Bremsstrahlung x-rays for 120 kVp is shown before passing through the beam filter, which shifts the average energies of the x-rays from one-third to one-half of the maximum energy possible.

In CT, the x-ray tube voltage ranges from 100 kVp to 140 kVp, with 120 kVp being the most commonly used tube voltage. Of the tube voltages greater than 100 kVp, 120 kVp typically is the chosen voltage in majority of the CT protocols because a tube voltage of approximately 120 kVp yields x-ray energy sufficient to penetrate most parts of the anatomy, including shoulder and pelvic areas. The larger the patient, the greater the tube voltage required to penetrate the thickest portion of the anatomy. There are certain protocols that use a lower tube voltage, such as

80 kVp. According to fundamentals of x-ray imaging, it is shown that the subject contrast is high at lower tube voltage, with increased skin absorption. Increasing the voltage decreases subject contrast but reduces skin entrance exposure. For pediatric protocols, it has been shown that the use of lower voltage has the advantage of lowering the overall radiation dose with minimal reduction in subject contrast. This is true especially with protocols in which iodine contrast is used. Because iodine has an absorption capability (K-edge) of approximately 80 keV, the anatomy containing iodine contrast will be greatly enhanced when scanned at lower voltage. The rule of thumb for determining the average energy of the x-ray beam is one-third to one-half of peak tube voltage (kVp). This relationship is true with the kVp ranges encountered in routine CT protocols.

Keeping all scan parameters constant and only changing tube voltage results in increase in the radiation dose to the patient. For example,

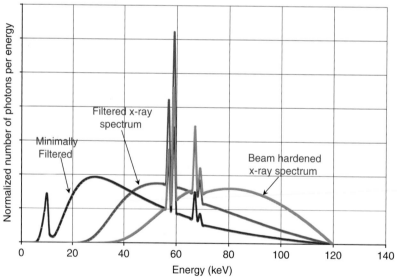

Figure 5.3. X-ray spectrum for tube voltage peak of 120 kVp is hardened by passing through different filter materials. The purpose of filtration is to remove low-energy x-rays (soft x-rays) before they enter the patient. Low-energy x-rays do not contribute to image formation but are absorbed on the patient skin surface. **A:** Minimal filtration provided by the x-ray tube window absorbs low energy soft x-rays. **B:** Filters such as aluminum (5–10 mm) further harden the x-ray beam. The average energy of x-ray beam is usually one-third of the maximum tube voltage; however, after filtration, the average energy is shifted closer to half of the maximum tube voltage. **C:** X-ray spectrum after passing through 30 cm of tissue-equivalent material.

when voltage is increased from 120 to 140, the radiation dose (described by $CTDI_{vol}$; details can be found in chapter on radiation dose) increases by a factor of ~1.4 and decreasing to 80 kVp reduces dose by approximately 2.2 times. The trade-off is the increased noise with lower voltage, as shown in Figure 5.4. At lower voltages, with increased attenuation of x-rays by varying tissues, the image contrast increases with lower tube voltage such as with bone, iodinated contrast agents, or metals. This is useful for scanning newborn and infants and thin patients where lower voltages are desired. Shown in Figure 5.5 are simulated abdominal images with identical mAs factors; however, the tube voltage is changed from 135 to 100 kVp. The corresponding gain in dose is represented along with the image noise, which tends to increase with lower kVp. The relationship between image quality, radiation dose, and kVp settings is quite complex and is important to understand to optimize scan protocols.

Key Points. A few key points about tube voltage are as follows: (a)For most CT applications, kVp is usually set at 120; (b) for thin patients and infants, kVp such as 80 and 100 has beneficial effects in reducing radiation dose and enhancing image contrast; and (c) For obese patients, it is advantageous to scan at greater kVp to penetrate thicker portion of the anatomy.

Tube Current and mAs. Tube current (mA) impacts the amount of x-rays produced in the x-ray tube. The product of tube current and scan time (s) is *milliamperes second* (mAs). Both mA and mAs have a linear impact on radiation dose in CT. The greater the mAs the greater the radiation dose to the patient. Also, the mAs impacts CT image noise linearly but inversely. With all other technical factors kept same, if the mAs is lowered, the radiation dose is lowered. However, the CT image becomes grainy and noisy and vice-versa (see Chapter 7). The effect of mAs on patient radiation dose is readily seen by changing mAs values in a protocol, which is reflected in the changing radiation dose ($CTDI_{vol}$) values (see Chapter 7 on radiation dose for details on dose descriptors). Because $CTDI_{vol}$ is readily accessible at the CT console, one can change mAs to

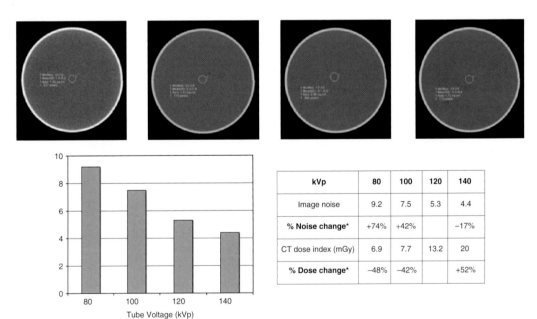

kVp	80	100	120	140
Image noise	9.2	7.5	5.3	4.4
% Noise change*	+74%	+42%		−17%
CT dose index (mGy)	6.9	7.7	13.2	20
% Dose change*	−48%	−42%		+52%

Figure 5.4. Effect of tube voltage on image noise and radiation dose are examined on CT images of a water phantom. All scan parameters are kept similar (such as tube current at 200 mA) and only tube voltage (kVp) is varied. Because 120 kVp is the most commonly used tube voltage, percent changes in image noise and radiation dose for other tube voltages are compared with those of 120-kVp images. Image noise decreases with increasing kVp; however, the radiation dose increases.

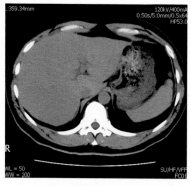
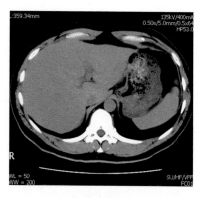

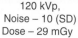

120 kVp,
Noise – 10 (SD)
Dose – 29 mGy

135 kVp,
Noise – 8 (SD)
Dose – 37 mGy

Figure 5.5. Effect of tube voltage (kVp) on image quality and radiation dose is demonstrated for simulated abdominal images at 120 kVp and 135 kVp, respectively. An increase of 12% in kVp results in an decrease of nearly 25% in image noise; however, the radiation dose increases by nearly 27%. Proper selection of tube voltage depends on the desired image quality required for proper diagnosis.

understand how it impacts the dose. In fact, among all the scan parameters, the most efficient way to reduce patient radiation dose is by lowering the tube current. With the demand for faster scans and thinner slices, the tube current is set very high (800 mA) in certain cardiac protocols. The use of high tube current setting becomes possible as the result of advances in x-ray tube technology.

Certain CT manufacturers use the concept of *effective mAs* during helical scanning. Effective mAs is the ratio of mAs to pitch and not simply the product of mA and scan time as described in the previous paragraph. To compensate for the

decrease in image noise, the mA is increased whenever pitch is increased (Table 5.1). For example: with effective mAs of 200, with scan time and all other scan factors held constant there can be many combinations of mA and pitch, such as if the pitch is increased to 1.5, mA is raised to 300 mA to maintain same image noise, similarly if the pitch is decreased to 0.75, the mA is lowered to 150 mA.

Scan Time and Gantry Time. Scan time is defined as the time during which the x-rays are *ON* during a single rotation of the x-ray tube inside the CT gantry. Normally, the x-ray tube is

Table 5.1	Relationship between effective mAs, mAs, pitch, and radiation dose		
Pitch	**mAs per rotation**	**Effective mAs**	**CTDI$_{vol}$**[a]
For constant mAs			
Axial	100	100	1.9
0.5	100	200	2.0
1	100	100	1.0
1.5	100	67	0.67
For constant mAs			
Axial scan	100	100	1.0
0.5	50	100	1.0
1	100	100	1.0
1.5	150	100	1.0

[a] Radiation dose descriptor discussed in detail in Chapter 7.

ON during the entire 360-degree rotation of the x-ray tube around the patient and is defined as *full rotation* (Fig. 5.6A). The demand for greater temporal resolution as in cardiac CT scans are driving the MDCT technology to develop faster and faster scan rotation time. One of the advantages of faster scan time is fewer motion artifacts, especially with rapidly moving organ such as heart. The scan time for reconstructing a CT image can be further reduced by limiting the x-ray *ON* time to only half of gantry rotation plus the fan angle (partial scan) rather than the entire 360-degree rotation (Fig. 5.6B). Also, with dual-source CT (DSCT) scanners, the temporal resolution is further improved by the use of data corresponding to quarter of the gantry rotation time for each of the two x-ray tubes (more details on DSCT can be found in later chapters; Fig. 5.6C). Scan times have dramatically decreased from 5 to 1 s in the first decade of the CT invention but decreased much slower through the second decade. In MDCT scanners it is now possible to achieve scan times below 300 milliseconds and, with partial scans, the scan time can be further lowered to less than 200 ms. Shorter scan time also enables to scan longer anatomy or shorter total scan time.

Scan times in CT has been dramatically decreasing over time (Fig. 5.7). In the past few years, the scan times have become even lower than half-a-second (500 ms) to less than 300 ms, almost reaching physical limitation in terms of gantry rotation. Faster scan time creates high centrifugal force on components inside the CT gantry. With scan time less than 500 ms, nearly 2–15 G forces are created inside the gantry during scan time, comparably higher than high speed aircrafts which yields 2–3 G forces. This poses a challenge for further reduction in scan time. The growing demand for greater temporal resolution has been the motivating force for CT manufacturers to consider dual x-ray tubes and there are currently researches underway to use more than two x-ray tubes.

When selecting a scan time, the user should make certain that the patient has adequate breath-holding capability and that the entire CT scan can be completed within the breath-holding time. If not, artifacts caused by breathing irregularity can impinge on the image quality in 3D images. In such case, scanning should be performed during shallow breathing, as in case of children or patients with breathing problem. This is especially important in hybrid scanners such as positron emission tomography (PET)-CT and single-photon emission computed tomography (SPECT)-CT (see Chapter 9 for more details).

Pitch. The concept of pitch was introduced with single-row detector helical CT (SDCT) scanners. During helical CT scanning, the patient

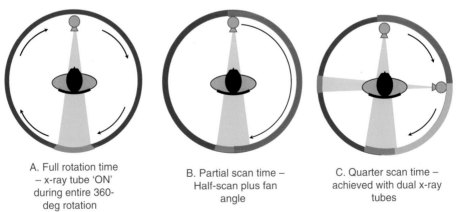

A. Full rotation time – x-ray tube 'ON' during entire 360-deg rotation

B. Partial scan time – Half-scan plus fan angle

C. Quarter scan time – achieved with dual x-ray tubes

Figure 5.6. Scan time is defined as the x-ray *ON* time during a single rotation of the x-ray tube inside the CT gantry rotation. **A:** Full rotation implies that the x-ray tube is *ON* during the entire 360 deg rotation. **B:** Partial scan implies x-ray tube is *ON* only for half of the gantry rotation time. **C:** Quarter scan time achieved with two x-ray tubes, each tube is *ON* for only quarter of the gantry rotation time.

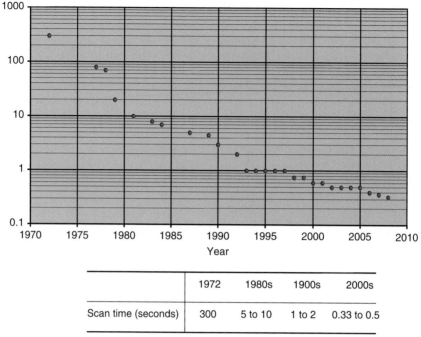

	1972	1980s	1900s	2000s
Scan time (seconds)	300	5 to 10	1 to 2	0.33 to 0.5

Figure 5.7. Scan times (full rotation) from the time of CT invention since 1972 have dramatically decreased during the years. Scan times on the order of less than 0.4 s or 400 ms are achieved in 64-row MDCT scanners.

table is transported through the gantry while the x-ray tube is continuously rotating around the patient yielding a spiral or helix data path. The *pitch* is defined as the ratio of the table feed per *gantry rotation to the x-ray beam width*. With the x-ray beam width given by W (in millimeter) and the table increment per gantry rotation defined as I (in millimeter), pitch is defined as:

$$Pitch = \frac{I}{W}$$

If the table feed is same as the x-ray beam width, it yields, a pitch = 1. This is same as sequential scan with table translated by increment of slice thickness, also known as abutted slices. The beam width in SDCT is the simply the slice width set at the time of CT scanning. With the introduction MDCT scanners, CT manufacturers defined pitch in different ways. Initially, terms such as *detector pitch, collimator pitch, slice pitch, volume pitch,* and so forth were introduced. This resulted in a lot of confusion earlier because the relationship between pitch, radia-

tion dose, and image quality were well established with SDCT and varying pitch definition would not confine to early definitions (Fig. 5.8). To distinguish the variation in pitch values, it is important to understand the following definitions of pitch.

Detector Pitch or Slice Pitch or Volume Pitch. Detector pitch is defined as ratio of table feed per gantry rotation to width of a single DAS channel width.

$$Detector\,Pitch = \frac{I}{T}$$

where T is the width of the single DAS channel. Typical values are 4, 6, 12, 18, and so on.

Beam Pitch or Collimator Pitch or Pitch Factor. It is similar to the pitch defined earlier in SDCT and is defined as the ratio of table feed per gantry rotation to the total x-ray beam width.

$$Beam\,Pitch = \frac{I}{W}$$

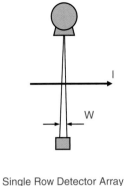

$$\text{Pitch} = \frac{I}{W}$$

$$\text{Detector Pitch} = \frac{I}{T}$$

$$\text{Beam Pitch} = \frac{I}{W}$$

$$\text{Beam Pitch} = \frac{\text{Detector Pitch}}{N}$$

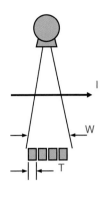

Single Row Detector Array
(SDCT)

Multiple Row Detector Array
(MDCT)

I - Table travel (mm)/rotation
W - Beam width (mm)

T - Single data acquisition channel width (mm)
N - Number of active data acquisition channels

$$\text{Radiation dose } \alpha \ \frac{I}{\text{Pitch}}$$

Figure 5.8. Illustration shows the concept pitch and other definitions introduced during the early times of MDCT scanners. Pitch is defined as the ratio of table travel per gantry rotation to the total x-ray beam width and is applicable across all type of helical CT scanners. Variations in the definition of pitch, such as detector pitch and beam pitch (same as pitch), applicable to MDCT scanners are also shown. In general, the radiation dose during helical scans varies inversely with pitch (From Mahesh M. Search for Isotropic Resolution in CT from Conventional through Multiple-Row Detector. *RadioGraphics* 2002;22:949–962, with permission.)

It is related to detector pitch as follows:

$$\text{Beam Pitch} = \frac{\text{Detector Pitch}}{N} = \frac{I}{N*T} = \frac{I}{W} = \text{Pitch}$$

where N is the number of DAS channels and T is the width of each DAS channel. Table 5.2 examines the relationship between table feed, detector pitch, and pitch for various MDCT detector configurations.

With international agreement (IEC) in place since 2003, currently all CT manufacturers are required to concur with the single definition of

Table 5.2	Relationship between pitch, detector pitch, and table speed for different MDCT configurations		
Table speed, mm/rotation	**MDCT configurations (N×T), mm**	**Detector pitch**	**Pitch[a]**
3.75	4 × 1.25	3	0.75
7.5	4 × 1.25	6	1.5
18	16 × 0.75	24	1.5
24	24 × 1.2	20	0.83
24	64 × 0.5	48	0.75
Most cardiac CT protocols (retrospectively gated) are performed at low pitch			
8	64 × 0.5	16	0.25
8	16 × 1.5	5.3	0.33
2	16 × 0.5	4	0.25

[a] Pitch equals the ratio of table speed to product of N and T.

pitch, defined as the ratio of table travel to total x-ray beam width. Adopting the usage of common definition of pitch is advantageous because it is applicable equally to both SDCT and MDCT scanners and eliminates confusion existing between the relationship of radiation dose and various definitions of pitch.

The Radiation Dose Is Inversely Proportional to the Pitch. Therefore, greater the pitch value means lower the radiation dose and vice-versa. The relationship between pitch and spatial resolution in the longitudinal direction depends on the type of interpolation algorithms selected during image reconstruction and is discussed in earlier chapter 3.

In summary, pitch greater than one (P > 1), implies extended imaging and reduced patient dose with lower axial spatial resolution. Pitch less than one (P < 1), implies overlapping and higher patient dose with higher axial spatial resolution. Pitch = 1 implies contiguous slice similar to sequential step-and-shoot scan. For example, 10-mm slice thickness with 10-mm slice interval.

Pitch values typically ranged from 0.2 to 1.5 for the various CT protocols, depending on the desired spatial resolution and concern for radiation dose. For routine abdominal imaging, a pitch greater than one is shown to be quite adequate in terms of image quality with added advantage of reduced radiation dose. For protocols that demand high spatial and temporal resolution, a pitch less than one (P < 1) are used, however this translates to greater patient dose. In fact these are the reasons why certain cardiac CT protocols, such as helical CT angiography procedures, demand pitch values as low as 0.2 to 0.4, translating into higher doses. Pitch variations with regard to heart rates, type of reconstruction algorithms and other factors are discussed in detail in chapter on cardiac CT.

Pitch is set for the entire scan, but options are available to vary pitch with regard to patient anatomy or organ's status. Concepts such as variable pitch or dynamic pitch are now possible with MDCT scanners. With this option, pitch can be varied automatically during the scans adjusting for the heart rate, and so forth.

Key Points. A few key points about pitch are as follows: (a) it is inversely proportional to radiation dose; (b) pitch > 1 means extended imaging of tissues/organs and, therefore, lower patient dose; and (c) pitch < 1 means overlapping of tissues/organs and, therefore, higher patient dose.

Scan Length. The length of the anatomy covered in a particular CT scan constitutes the scan length. The user then prescribes the scan length on the scout image. The radiation exposure to patient increases with increasing scan length. As shown in the CT dose report (Fig. 5.9), the scan length per CT scan can be determined by simply dividing the dose-length-product (DLP) and $CTDI_{vol}$. For a particular scan protocol, $CTDI_{vol}$ remains constant, and therefore scan length influences the DLP. Because scan length affects the total dose to the patient, it is important to prescribe the scan length as close as possible to the area of interest but still make sure that the desired anatomy is not missed. Proper patient instructions, experienced CT technologists, and use of standard CT protocols will help to minimize the instances of selecting excessive scan region. Even then, in helical CT acquisition, the ramp up and ramp down of the helical scan can result in additional exposure at the beginning and at the end of the helical CT scans. This is shown in Fig. 5.10: the beam width is well defined in a sequential scan compared with a helical scan, and the x-ray beam width is larger, resulting in larger scan length compared with the helical scan mode. This has direct impact on overall radiation dose to the patients. Some CT manufacturers are beginning to introduce *adaptive shielding* or *dynamic collimation* to block extraneous radiation during the ramp up or ramp down to patient during helical CT scan. In such cases, the collimation is partly closed at the beginning of the helical scan, opens during the first rotation and at the end again closes during the last rotation.

Secondary Scan Parameters

Scan Field of View. Scan field of view (SFOV) is defined as the region in the CT gantry within which the anatomy is included in the image reconstruction. Typically, the SFOV is

Exam Description: PET/CT RESTAGING OVARI					
		Dose Report			
Series	Type	Scan Range (mm)	CTDIvol (mGy)	DLP (mGy-cm)	Phantom cm
1	Scout	–	–	–	–
2	Helical	110.500–1867.240	7.89	712.36	Body 32
			Total Exam DLP:	712.36	

Total mAs 17696	Total DLP 2419					
	Scan	KV	mAs / ref.	CTDIvol	DLP	TI	cSL
Patient Position H-SP						
Topogram	1	120				7.8	0.6
ARTERIAL	2	120	400	28.67	920	0.33	0.6
VENOUS	3	120	400	28.69	1499	0.33	0.6

Figure 5.9. CT dose reports lists both CTDI$_{vol}$ and DLP. The ratio of DLP and CTDI$_{vol}$ provides the scan length. Increasingly, all MDCT manufacturers are providing this information that can be saved as part of study and can be accessed remotely for analysis. As always, the CTDI$_{vol}$ is the dose descriptor measured on standard size circular phantoms. **A:** Dose report for a PET-CT study yielding a scan length of 90 cm. **B:** Dose report for an abdominal study yielding a total scan length of 32 cm during arterial phase and 52 cm during venous phase respectively.

less than the gantry opening (50–55 cm in diameter) and that is why sometimes certain anatomical regions (such as shoulder or pelvis) appear to be chopped-off in the reconstructed image. Although the CT gantry opening is 70 cm in diameter, the actual SFOV is around 50–55 cm (Fig. 5.11). For this reason, the object to be scanned should be positioned at the center of the gantry aperture, also known as the isocenter. Care should be taken to position the object of interest at isocenter in the CT gantry; if not, the image quality can be degraded and so is the radiation dose to the patient. In Figure 5.12, a patient positioned above the isocenter and closer to the

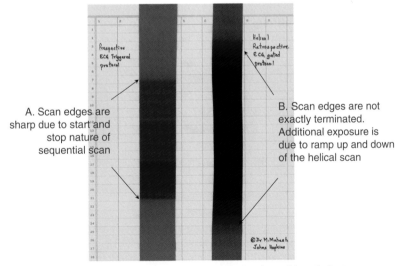

A. Scan edges are sharp due to start and stop nature of sequential scan

B. Scan edges are not exactly terminated. Additional exposure is due to ramp up and down of the helical scan

Figure 5.10. Scan lengths are closer to the specified/indicated length during sequential CT scans (**A**) compared to helical CT scans (**B**). During helical CT scan, the actual scan length is slightly greater than specified in the topograph. As shown, the ramp up and ramp down of the helical scan can yield an additional exposure both at the beginning and end of the CT scans.

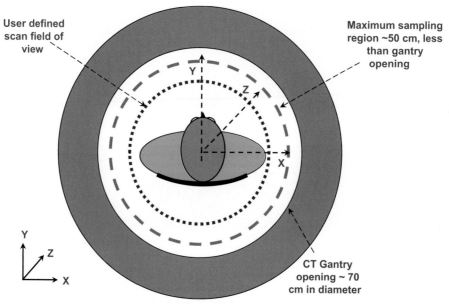

Figure 5.11. Schematic diagram of a CT gantry illustrating that the maximum sampling region (∼50 cm in diameter) is less than the physical gantry opening (∼70 cm in diameter). The user-defined scan field of view is within the maximum sampling region. Also illustrated is the x–y plane defined as the in-plane or axial plane and the z-axis, indicating the longitudinal direction.

x-ray tube results in increased patient radiation dose during scout scan, whereas a patient positioned below the isocenter and away from the x-ray tube results in noisy image. Positioning of patients to isocenter is important to obtain optimal image quality and dose. Especially in MDCT scanner with dose modulation techniques, patient positioning at the gantry isocenter becomes even more critical because dose-modulation techniques assumes patient to be at isocenter and any deviation from that position can instruct the scanner to increase dose markedly.

Also, in MDCT, as the x-ray beam width increases (as with 16 or 64 or 320 MDCT scanners) so do the cone-beam artifacts. The cone beam artifacts are less severe at the isocenter

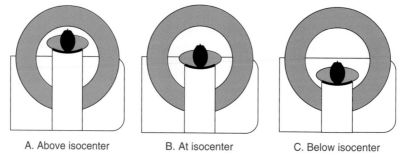

Figure 5.12. Patient positioning in the CT gantry is important in terms of image quality and radiation dose. These three cases demonstrate the significance of positioning the patient at isocenter and how it can impact image quality and radiation dose. **A:** The patient is positioned too high above the isocenter, which yields greater dose during scout scan and suboptimal image quality for axial scans. **B:** The patient is positioned correctly at the isocenter, yielding optimal image quality and radiation dose. **C:** The patient is positioned too low below the isocenter, yielding low dose during scout scan but suboptimal images during axial scans.

compared with those at the periphery of the SFOV. Therefore, in CT it is critical that the examined region is positioned as close as possible to the isocenter of the gantry. This is often verified by performing a quick scan or a target scan before starting the CT series. The positioning of the patient at isocenter becomes even more critical when dose modulation techniques are applied (for more details, see Chapter 8). Improper positioning can result in increased mAs settings and, therefore, an increased radiation dose to the patient, especially when scanning with dose-modulation techniques.

Beam Width or Beam Collimation. Beam width or beam collimation implies the total x-ray beam exiting the x-ray tube that is incident upon the patient. It is defined at the isocenter of the CT scanner. In SDCT, the beam-width is same as the slice width. However, in MDCT, the beam width is the product of the number of DAS channels and the thickness of each DAS channels. Therefore, the beam width is 1 mm for detector configuration of 2 × 0.5 mm, 4 mm for 4 × 1 mm, 10 mm for 4 × 2.5 mm, 20 mm for 32 × 0.75 mm, and 40 mm for 64 × 0.625 mm, respectively (Fig. 5.13). Larger beam-widths (128 mm with 256 × 0.5 mm and 160 mm with 320 × 0.5 mm) have a unique advantage in covering large area enabling wider anatomical coverage, there by scanning entire organ such as heart in a single gantry rotation.

The choices of larger total beam widths (N×T) in MDCT scanners have resulted in faster and volumetric scanning a reality. The beam width or beam collimation is defined with reference to scan plane at the isocenter of the CT gantry. Therefore, for scanners with larger number of detectors, a beam width such as 12.8 cm or 16.0 mm is found at the isocenter and the beam width is smaller away from isocenter as the result of cone beam. In Figure 5.14, the beam width of a 64 and 320 MDCT scanner at isocenter and 16 cm away (head phantom size) from isocenter are shown. With large coverage detectors, the cone beam effect needs to be carefully evaluated since the beam coverage is not the same at the surface and center of a phantom or patient (Fig. 5.14). With the scan parameters being same, increasing beam width, has markedly reduced the scan time from 4-slice MDCT scanner to 64-slice MDCT scanner (Fig. 5.15).

Slice Width/Slice Thickness/Section Width. Slice width or slice thickness or section width is the thickness of the reconstructed CT image. The term slice width is followed in this

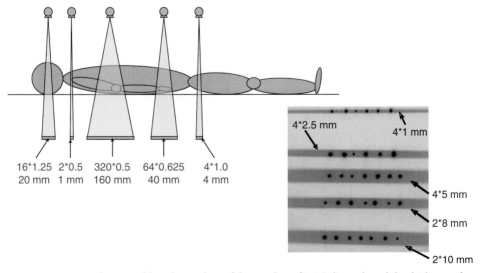

Figure 5.13. X-ray beam width is the product of the number of DAS channels and the thickness of each DAS channel. The beam width is defined at the isocenter of the CT gantry and is illustrated for various MDCT detector configurations. X-ray beam widths measured at isocenter also are shown.

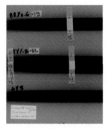

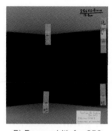

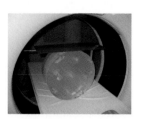

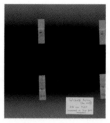

A) Beam width for 64 MDCT @ isocenter (24*1.2 mm)

B) Beam width for 256 MDCT @ isocenter (256*0.5 mm)

C) Recording media placed on top of body phantom (32 cm in dia meter)

D) Beam width for 256 MDCT @ 16 cm from isocenter (256*0.5 mm)

Figure 5.14. X-ray beam widths measured at isocenter for Siemens Sensation 64 MDCT scanner (defined maximum beam width is $24 \times 1.2 = 28.8$ mm) and for Toshiba 256 MDCT scanner (defined maximum beam width is $256 \times 0.5 = 128$ mm). Also shown is the beam width at 16 cm from isocenter (on top surface of a standard CT body phantom of 32 cm in diameter), which is much smaller (90 to 100 mm) than the defined beam width due to cone beam effect.

book to imply the reconstructed CT image width. In MDCT, the slice width is influenced by the individual DAS channel width, pitch, and the type of reconstruction algorithm. Slice width is always equal to or greater than the DAS channel width. In helical scan mode, it varies in a complex fashion from 100% to 130% of the DAS

channel width when pitch is increased from 1 to 2 and with certain type of interpolation algorithms used in image reconstruction. Slice width cannot be smaller than the DAS channel width. In fact, this is one of the reasons why there has been rapid improvement in detector technology to develop thinner and thinner detector assem-

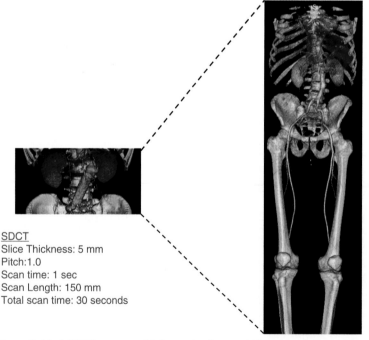

MDCT (4 slice)
Slice Thickness: 3 mm
Pitch:1.5
Scan time: 0.5 sec
Scan Length: 1000 mm
Total scan time: 30 seconds

SDCT
Slice Thickness: 5 mm
Pitch:1.0
Scan time: 1 sec
Scan Length: 150 mm
Total scan time: 30 seconds

MDCT (16 slice)
Slice Thickness: 3 mm
Pitch:1.5
Scanning time: 0.5 sec
Scan Length: 1000 mm
Total scan time: ~10 seconds

Figure 5.15. MDCT scanners with increasing beam width can cover large anatomy in short duration. For equivalent scan parameters, shown are the comparisons of anatomical coverage and scan duration between single-row detector CT (SDCT), four-slice, and 16-slice MDCT scanners. For a scan time of 30 s, an SDCT scanner covers 150 mm, whereas the four-slice MDCT scanner covers approximately 1000 mm. Scan time to cover 1000 mm is further decreased to less than 10 s in 16-slice MDCT scanner (From Toshiba Medical Systems, with permission).

bly so as to obtain thin slices for improved three-dimensional image reconstruction.

Before MDCT, in single-detector spiral CT (SDCT) the slice width is same as the x-ray beam width or beam collimation. The slice width then varied as the beam collimation, pitch and the type of interpolation algorithm used in the image reconstruction. Even then, the slice width is always equal to or greater than the beam collimation.

Reconstruction Algorithms (Kernels). Reconstruction algorithms are computer programs applied to reconstruct raw CT projection data and have unique role in CT image quality. The selection of reconstruction algorithms always involves trade-off between spatial and contrast resolution. Users can choose from a range of reconstruction algorithms specifically developed for specific anatomy or function. In general, the algorithms are classified as *very smooth, smooth, medium smooth, sharp, and ultra sharp* depending on the desired image quality. Algorithms are also grouped according to the type of scan such as head, body, children, and special applications.

The selection of reconstruction algorithm always involves a trade-off between spatial and contrast resolution. A high-resolution reconstruction algorithm provides high-resolution CT images but yields greater image noise and often introduces edge-enhanced artifacts. Soft or smooth algorithm reduces image noise but also reduces sharpness. Often for viewing images from obese patients, where the image noise is greater due to few x-ray photons reaching the detectors, using smoothing algorithms reduces image noise but not degrade spatial resolution. In Figure 5.16, the image noise measured at the same location on the CT images of a water phantom reconstructed with various reconstruction algorithms shows the degradation of image noise with sharper reconstruction algorithms.

Increasing computing capability in MDCT scanners provides an opportunity to reconstruct multiple image sets with different reconstruction algorithms from one set of raw data. In fact, it is now convenient to acquire raw data with thinnest slice as possible, to reconstruct high-quality three-dimensional images and, at the same time, additional reconstructions with smoothing algorithms will allow the user to visualize less noisy CT image for interpretation. In MDCT with increasing number of detectors, the mantra is *"to scan thin and reconstruct thick slices as desired"*. Because raw data are obtained once and different image sets can be reconstructed with various reconstruction algorithms, it has no direct impact on patient radiation dose. Figure 5.17 shows how the image quality on abdominal CT images varies with different reconstruction algorithms with sharpest algorithms yielding the highest image noise and highest spatial resolution. The choice of the reconstruction algorithms depends on the type of visualization required for interpretation. For example, to detect low-contrast objects such as small liver lesions, normally smooth algorithms are chosen.

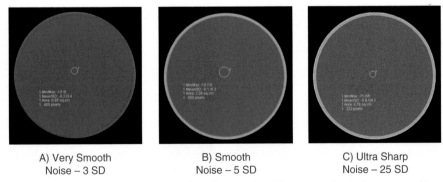

A) Very Smooth
Noise – 3 SD

B) Smooth
Noise – 5 SD

C) Ultra Sharp
Noise – 25 SD

Figure 5.16. Effect of reconstruction algorithms on the CT image quality is demonstrated in water phantom images. CT images obtained on 64-slice MDCT scanner are reconstructed with (**A**) very smooth, (**B**) smooth, and (**C**) ultra-sharp reconstruction algorithms. The image noise increases sharply with use of the ultra-sharp reconstruction algorithm.

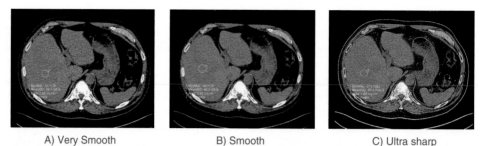

A) Very Smooth   B) Smooth   C) Ultra sharp

Figure 5.17. Effect of reconstruction algorithms on the CT image quality is demonstrated in abdominal images. CT abdominal images obtained on 64-slice MDCT scanner are reconstructed with **(A)** very smooth, **(B)** smooth, and **(C)** ultra-sharp reconstruction algorithms. The image noise increases sharply with use of the ultra-sharp reconstruction algorithm.

On the other hand, to detect defect in the lung or temporal bone, sharp reconstruction algorithms are chosen. Judicious selection of reconstruction algorithm and mAs will help reduce the radiation dose. In fact, research efforts are under way to apply iterative reconstruction algorithms to CT data, which has a good potential to reduce radiation dose and to reduce image noise by an order of magnitude.

Reconstruction Interval. The reconstruction interval is the distance between the reconstructed images in the z-direction. It defines the degree of overlap between reconstructed axial images. Reconstruction interval is also known as *reconstruction increment, reconstruction index or spacing.* It is independent of x-ray beam collimation or image thickness (slice width) and has no effect on scan time or patient exposure. When the reconstruction interval is smaller than the slice thickness, the images are created with

an overlap. The reason for decreased reconstruction interval (or increased overlap) is to reduce partial volume effect and to improve z-axis resolution, especially for three-dimensional and multiple planar reconstruction (MPR) images. If the reader is making a diagnosis based on only axial images, reconstruction interval is not an issue. In fact, in certain protocols, large reconstruction interval yields fewer numbers of images that must be reconstructed and interpreted. This is especially the case in high-resolution chest CT protocol, where few thin slices are scanned or reconstructed for interpretation (Fig. 5.18). However, the main disadvantage is that they do not provide optimum lesion detection and in fact yield lower detection rates. With MDCT scanners, high-resolution (HR) CT protocols are less used; instead they are replaced with thin detector acquisition through the entire chest minimizing misdetection of any pathology at the burden of increased radiation dose.

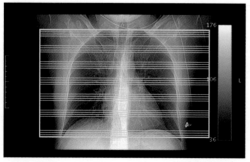

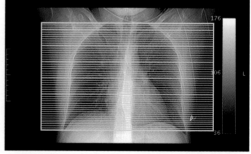

Figure 5.18. During HRCT protocols, the patient's chest region is scanned in thin-slice acquisition mode with large scan intervals resulting in few thin slices. However, in MDCT scanners, HRCT protocols are replaced with thin-slice acquisition throughout the chest region to minimize any type of misdetection of pathology. The radiation dose estimation with HRCT is relatively lower (1–2 mSv) compared with a regular chest CT (5–7 mSv) that obtains thin slices throughout the chest region.

Overlapping axial images results in a relatively large number of images but also can result in improved lesion visibly in MPR and 3D images without increasing the patient dose (Fig. 5.19). In fact, physicians are reading MPR and 3D images; this is especially true for cardiac CT. For routine MPR and 3D applications, a 30% image overlap is generally sufficient (1-mm slice with 0.7-mm reconstruction interval). It should be recognized that too much overlap results in a large number of images, increases reconstruction time, can result in longer interpretation periods, and can put undue strain on image handling overhead costs (image transfer, image display, image archive, etc) with no significant gain in image quality.

Display Field of View. The display field of view (DFOV) is determined by the need for displaying desired region of interest. For example, in cardiac CT, although the entire chest region is scanned, the DFOV is limited to the heart region, omitting portion of the chest from display. A constant DFOV instead should be used throughout the scanned body region to allow for multiplanar reformatting or three-dimensional reconstruction or fusing CT images with images obtained from other modalities, such as PET-CT. In such cases, the DFOV should be based on the largest portion of the scanned region. For small objects, the size of the DFOV can be reduced further to improve image quality. This is especially true with the scanning of temporal bones or neck, where the DFOV is chosen to correspond to the object size, that is, by zooming to the area of interest.

The DFOV is always less than or equal to the SFOV. When a certain region in the SFOV needs to be visualized closer, often magnifying the regions is sufficient. However, magnifying too much can deteriorate image resolution (Fig. 5.20). On many occasion the DFOV is chosen to be smaller than the SFOV view with the purpose of displaying certain region into the entire image matrix, as in case of cardiac CT. The process of displaying smaller region on the entire image matrix is called *zooming* and is expressed by *zooming factor*, which is defined as the ratio of the SFOV to DFOV. It has an advantage over magnification in that it provides improved resolution (Fig. 5.20). In such cases, selecting a smaller region and

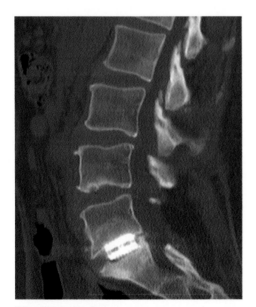

Slice Thickness 2 mm
Reconstruction Interval 5 mm

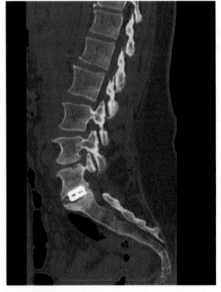

Slice Thickness 2 mm
Reconstruction Interval 1 mm

Figure 5.19. Sagittal reconstruction of lumbar spine axial images (2-mm slice thickness) with reconstruction intervals of 5 mm demonstrates significant loss in details compared with images with a 1-mm reconstruction intervals.

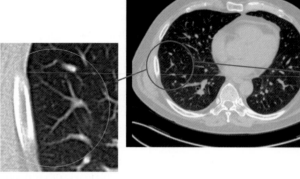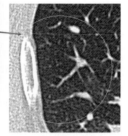

Magnification factor – 4
(400 mm DFOV)

Zoom factor - 4
(100 mm DFOV)

Figure 5.20. Zooming versus magnification concepts are illustrated in high-resolution chest CT image. High-resolution chest CT image magnified by a factor of four demonstrate loss of spatial resolution caused by pixilated image quality, whereas zooming by a factor four (field of view from 400 to 100 mm) demonstrates an increase in image sharpness and no loss in image detail. Zooming is advantageous over magnification in CT because spatial resolution loss is minimal; however, zooming results in image of smaller field of view.

reconstructing that particular smaller region can improve spatial resolution.

The reconstruction with the larger zoom factor often is used to exclude the influence of the image matrix. Therefore, if the zoom factor is equal to one, then the display field of view is the same as the scan field of view. The pixel size of the displayed image that influences the image resolution is given by the ratio of the display field of view and the number of pixels used. For example, if DFOV is 50 cm and the image matrix is 512 × 512 pixels, then the pixel size is equal to the 50 cm divided by 512 results to 0.1 cm or 1 mm pixel resolution respectively. To display smaller and smaller area, zoom factor is increased from 1 to 2. To diminish the influence of image matrix and improve spatial resolution, a zoom factor of 4 or more is often selected when details less than 0.5 mm is the target resolution which leads to decrease in DFOV. For example, decreasing DFOV from 50 cm to 20 cm and keeping same image matrix, the pixel resolution improves from 1 mm to 0.4 mm.

Although the SFOV is less than the gantry opening, certain MDCT manufacturers have begun to provide *extended SFOV* or *virtual SFOV* all the way to the CT gantry opening. This is especially the case with CT simulators used in radiation oncology, where patients are scanned before planning their radiation treatment. In these CT scanners, also called *large-bore* or *open-field gantry*, the image reconstruction process virtually recreates images that extends all the way to the gantry opening, even though the actual SFOV is less than the gantry opening.

CT Values, Uniformity, Contrast, and Linearity. CT values or CT numbers are defined by two fixed points, water and air. As discussed in the chapter 2, the x-ray absorption through tissues expressed as the attenuation values are mapped on to a gray scale and for convenience the individual voxel attenuation values are scaled to more convenient integers and normalized to voxel values containing water (μ_w). CT numbers are computed as:

$$CT\# = K \frac{\mu_m - \mu_w}{\mu_w}$$

where, μ_m is the measured attenuation of the material in the voxel and K (1000) is the scaling factor. The CT numbers are expressed as Hounsfield Units (HU). The attenuation coefficient of water is obtained during calibration of the CT machine. Voxels containing materials that attenuate more than water, for example, muscle tissue, liver, and bone, have positive CT numbers, whereas materials with less attenuation than water, such as lung or adipose tissues, have negative CT numbers. With the exception of water and air, which are pegged at 0 HU and –1000 HU, the CT numbers for a given material will vary with changes in the x-ray tube potential and from manufacturer to manufacturer.

For every CT scanner, the points for water and air are fixed using phantom measurements for each tube voltage and for each x-ray filtration choices available. In fact, it is required to check at regular intervals to ensure the CT values for water and air are within acceptable limits. The determination of CT number by scanning a water phantom is one of the fundamental requirements for daily quality control.

In addition to checking CT number of water on a regular basis, the CT number across the reconstructed image is measured to check the uniformity. The goal is to ensure homogeneity or uniformity across the entire cross section. CT number accuracy and uniformity are measured by the use of cylindrical water phantoms (Fig. 5.21). The tolerance for variation of CT numbers for water should be within the tolerance specified by the CT manufacturers. With increasing demand for maintaining CT image quality and radiation dose, several volunteer CT accreditation programs are available. According to one such CT accreditation program (American College of Radiology, Reston, VA), the CT number for water is required to be with in 0 ± 7 HU and the uniformity is required to be with ± 7 HU when measured from center to edge of a uniform water phantom.

Window Selection. The selection of proper window for image viewing critical for correct diagnosis is no longer an issue with MDCT. Earlier, users spent considerable amounts of time windowing the CT image for proper viewing of the CT image. There are many preset windows that user can select to display CT images in

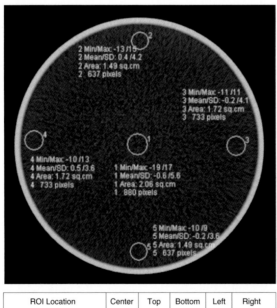

ROI Location	Center	Top	Bottom	Left	Right
Mean CT Number (HU)	−0.6	0.4	−0.2	0.5	−0.2
Deviation from center		−1.0	−0.4	−0.1	−0.4

Figure 5.21. CT number accuracy and uniformity is examined by measuring mean CT number at various locations on a homogeneous water phantom. The mean CT number for water should be close to 0 HU and acceptable limits for variation in CT number is often set to 0 ± 7 HU.

MDCT scanners and there is also option to adjust the window level manually.

The MDCT scanners have the capability of 4096 gray tones ($2^{12} = 4096$ level) to represent various density levels in HU. The monitor can display CT images with varying gray tones ranging from 256 to 4096, yet the human eye can discriminate approximately 20 shades of gray tones. Therefore, it is important to select the window setting to represent the density of the tissue of interest. Ideally, the window level (center) should be chosen close to the CT number of the primary structure of interest (for example, 40–50 HU for grey matter imaging). Next, the window width should be wide enough to capture all relevant structures but as narrow as possible. The window width influences image contrast. Narrow windows are useful for detecting changes in tissue characteristics in a small region, for example to detect changes in lung tissues. While window width may have to be increased for images that include both high-contrast and low contrast structures. A large window width decreases the visibility of image noise and may be useful for low-dose examinations in which local contrast is not critical.

Image Noise. For routine purposes, the image noise in CT is determined by the standard deviation of CT numbers in the select *region of interest* (ROI). Although there are more complicated formulas to estimate image noise, the first order estimation of image noise is simply the standard deviation of CT number in the select ROI (Fig. 5.22). Image noise defines the quality of the CT image as discussed elsewhere in this chapter and is influenced by variety of factors including kVp, mAs, reconstructed algorithms, slice thickness, and many other factors.

Efficiency. It is the ability of the CT system to detect or use all the x-ray photons exiting the patient. The efficiency has direct impact on patient dose and image quality. The overall efficiency of a CT system is more or less the product of the sensitivity of individual detector elements and geometric efficiency of the multiple detectors. The sensitivity of detector elements depends on the detector's absorption and conversion properties and usually is greater than

90%. It is also dependent on the type of materials used in the detector construction. Details about the type of detector materials and composition are often proprietary and are well guarded by manufacturers and only specify the efficiency in the manuals.

The efficiency can further be understood by examining two aspects. First, the absorption of x-ray photons by the narrow strips (septa) that are between the detector elements and do not contribute to final detector signal. Each multidetector elements are separated by narrow strips to avoid cross-talk between the elements and to absorb scatter radiation. This is often called the geometric efficiency and can be calculated by dividing the active area of the detector array by the total radiation area of the detector. Typical values range from 70% to 90% and tend to decrease with more number of detector elements.

Second is the efficiency of the x-ray beam utilization in the longitudinal axis, which is also called *geometric efficiency (Isometric detector)*. It is often defined as the fraction of the x-ray beam profile that hits the detector elements in the longitudinal direction. In MDCT, it is required to have roughly equal numbers of x-ray photons strike all active detectors in the z-direction to maintain similar image quality. This requirement means that the natural shadowing of the beam (penumbra) attributable to the finite-sized focal spot is intentionally positioned to strike outside of the active detector elements. This phenomenon called *overbeaming* results in a reduced longitudinal efficiency in MDCT. This was not the case in SDCT, where all the radiation including primary and penumbra reaching the detector was utilized in image formation resulting in maximum geometric efficiency (Fig. 5.23).

The reduction in longitudinal efficiency is especially true with first-generation MDCT scanners while scanning with protocols using few thin detectors, such as 4×0.5 mm or 4×1 mm. The width of the penumbra is fairly constant with each scanner, generally in the range of 1–3 mm. The proportion of radiation wasted relative to the overall width of the x-ray beam varies with the protocol used. If very thin images are required and the overall x-ray beam width is

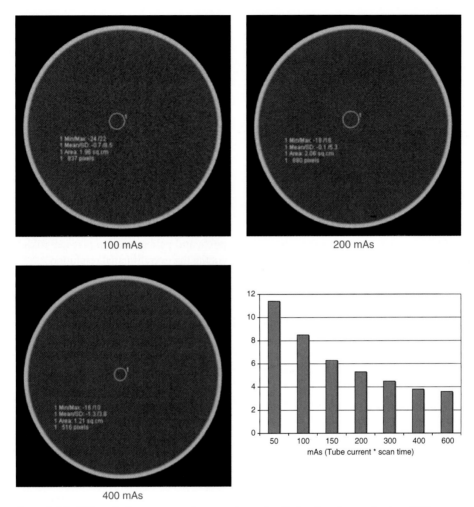

Figure 5.22. Effect of tube current on image noise and radiation dose is examined on CT images of a water phantom. All scan parameters are kept similar (such as tube voltage at 120 kVp), and only the mAs (tube current × scan time) is varied. Percent changes in image noise and radiation dose for other tube voltages are compared with those of 200 mAs images. Image noise decreases with increasing mAs and the radiation dose increases both changes occur in linear fashion.

small—5 mm (4 × 1.25 mm), for example—then the proportion of wasted x-rays could be 20–60% (resulting in a dose efficiency of 40–80%). If thin images are not required and a wider x-ray beam is used—20 mm (16 × 1.25 mm) for example—then the proportion of wasted x-rays would be 5–15% (resulting in a dose efficiency of 85–95%). In general, with increasing number of detector rows, the fraction of over beamed area to total detector areas decreases, and z-axis efficiency improves. Radiation dose increases markedly with narrowing beams and fewer active detector elements, but less so for wider beam and more detectors owing to improved geometry efficiency (Fig. 5.24).

Image Quality-Related Parameters

Resolution. Resolution in medical image demonstrates the imaging modality's ability to resolve objects close to each other (spatial resolution), distinguish objects from background (contrast resolution), or record events occurring within short duration (temporal resolution). In this section, spatial resolution and

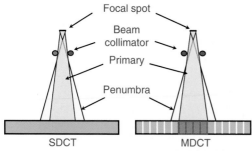

Figure 5.23. Geometric efficiency is defined as the fraction of x-ray beam that intercepts the detector elements in longitudinal direction. Geometric efficiency is optimal with SDCT because radiation from both the primary and penumbra region is used in image formation. On the other hand, to maintain uniformity across all the detector elements, radiation from penumbra region is excluded in the image formation. In MDCT, the penumbra region is intenionally positioned to strike outside the detector elements, resulting in overbeaming and therefore is associated with lower geometric efficiency.

spatial resolution has been historically high in axial plane (x–y plane) and with MDCT scanners; the z-axis resolution has also improved markedly. The achievement of isotropic resolution (axial and longitudinal resolution same) is one of the main goals of the technological development with MDCT scanners. There are number of factors that influence the spatial resolution in CT scanners. Among them, the key factors are x-ray focal spot size and shape, detector aperture, scanner geometry, and reconstruction algorithm. In addition, with MDCT scanners, the detector size in longitudinal direction, reconstruction algorithms, reconstruction intervals, pitch, and patient motion play key roles in influencing the overall spatial resolution.

In medical imaging, spatial resolution is typically specified as spatial frequencies and expressed in terms of line-pairs per centimeters (lp/cm) or line pairs per millimeters (lp/mm). Bar patterns often are the chosen tool for measuring spatial resolution. Bar patterns are patterns of various sizes finely etched in a sheet of high attenuation material (such as lead). A line pair is a pair of equally sized black and white bars. If the CT manufacturer specifies that the CT scanner has a spatial resolution capability of 1 lp/cm, it means that the scanner can resolve 1 line-pair that can fits in 1 centimeter of space, which means that each line is 0.5 cm or 5 mm in size. Therefore, a system with 1 lp/cm resolution has the capability to resolve objects of up to

contrast resolution in CT are discussed along with the factors affecting the resolution while temporal resolution is discussed in more detail in chapter 6 on cardiac CT.

Spatial Resolution. Spatial resolution is the ability to resolve or distinguish objects of certain size placed closed to each other. Spatial resolution in CT is often specified two ways, namely axial (x–y plane) and longitudinal (z-axis). The

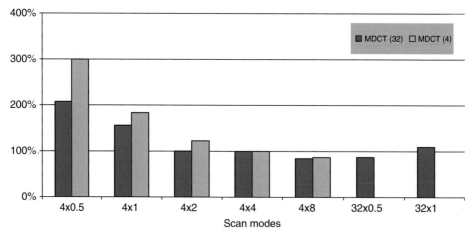

Figure 5.24. Radiation dose grows markedly with thin collimation and with few active detectors. Geometric efficiency is lower in the four-slice compared with 32-slice MDCT scanner.

0.5 cm or 5 mm placed closed to each other and any objects smaller than that size are not resolvable. Similarly, a scanner with 10 lp/cm spatial resolution has the capacity to resolve objects of up to 0.5 mm size objects placed close to each other.

Direct measurements with bar patterns are easily performed in a clinical setting and are relatively easy to interpret; however, their interpretation is subjective and depends on the viewing condition and interpretation. On the other hand, objective and quantitative determination of spatial resolution is determined using *modulation transfer function* (MTF). Although the MTF method is not easy and involves complex computer calculations, nevertheless, the CT manufacturer specified spatial resolution based on MTF method because it provides an objective assessment. MTF is defined as the ratio of the output modulation to input modulation. Basically, it is a way to measure how an image system (CT scanner) accepts the input information and transmits through the system (CT scanner) and creates the output image. Ideally, one desires to design an imaging system that has the capability to completely transfer the input infor-

mation (patient information) into output signal (CT image).

If the system can transfer all of the input information perfectly, then the MTF of that system is 1, which implies that the information is transferred completely with any degradation. On the other hand, if the system transfers information variably according to the characteristics of the object (e.g., size), then the MTF decreases and eventually reaches 0. MTF are expressed graphically with MTF values shown on the y-coordinate ranging from 0 to 1 and the spatial frequencies are depicted on the x-coordinates. A value of 0 implies that the output signal is completely degraded and 1 implies that the output signal (image) is as true as the input (scanned object). For an ideal imaging system, the MTF has a straight (Fig. 5.25) line and is independent of the input spatial frequency (Spatial frequency $\propto$ 1/object size). Practically, there is certain amount of degradation with any imaging method and therefore MTF curve decreases with increasing spatial frequencies (smaller objects) and eventually reaches 0, as shown in Figure 5.26. The point where the MTF reaches 0.2 is

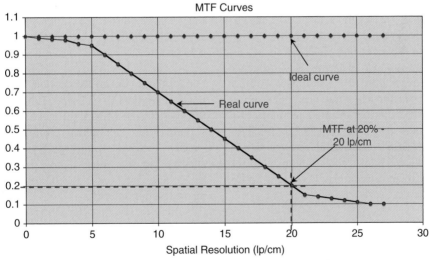

Figure 5.25. MTF demonstrates the ability of the spatial resolution of an imaging system. Indicated is **(A)** the ideal MTF curve capable of resolving objects of all different sizes with any degradation, whereas **(B)** the real MTF curves shows how the capability to resolve objects degrades with objects size becoming smaller. The performance of CT scanner is often specified by the spatial resolution corresponding to 0.2 values of MTF curve. It provides a uniform method to compare either various scanning parameters of a single CT scanner or compare different CT scanners for a single imaging parameter.

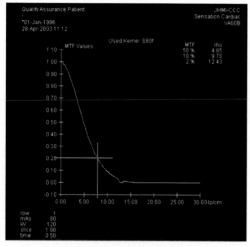

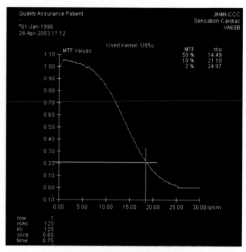

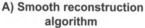

| A) Smooth reconstruction | B) Ultra-sharp |
| algorithm | reconstruction algorithm |

Figure 5.26. MTF curves demonstrate the capability of a MDCT scanner for two different reconstruction algorithms. **A:** MTF curve for smooth reconstruction algorithm yielding a spatial resolution on the order of 7.5 lp/cm (line-pairs per centimeter). **B:** MTF curve for ultra-sharp reconstruction algorithm, yielding a spatial resolution of 17 lp/cm at a cut-off MTF of 0.2.

often considered the limiting frequency for the CT scanner.

Performance data sheets provided by CT manufacturers often use 50%, 10%, and 0% MTF to indicate the frequencies (lp/cm) corresponding to the points on the MTF curves. The comparison of CT scanners for spatial resolution capability often is performed by measuring resolution at 20% or at 10% MTF.

There are number of factors that influence the spatial resolution in CT scanners. Among them the key factors are x-ray focal spot size and shape, detector aperture, scanner geometry, and reconstruction algorithm (Fig. 5.27). In addition, with MDCT scanners, the detector size in longitudinal direction, reconstruction intervals, pitch and patient motion play key role in influencing the overall spatial resolution.

Axial (x–y plane) Resolution. The axial resolution has always been high in CT and ranges from 5 to 20 lp/cm capability in resolving objects of 1 to 0.25 mm in size (Fig. 5.28). In comparison, conventional radiographic systems have an even greater resolution (40 to 200 lp/cm) with film-screen mammography (up to 200 lp/cm); yet, the many advantages of CT, including its ability to provide three-dimensional

images of three-dimensional objects (without superimposition of tissues) and superior contrast resolution, have trumped the use of CT (Table 5.3). Axial resolution is dependent on the DFOV and the image reconstruction matrix. For example, a 25-cm DFOV with 512 × 512 image matrix yields an axial resolution of 10 lp/cm or capability to resolve objects of up to 0.5 mm size.

Longitudinal (z-axis) Resolution. The longitudinal resolution in CT was simply the slice thickness before MDCT scanners. With MDCT scanners, the longitudinal resolution is influenced by the DAS channel width and in addition affected by the interpolation reconstruction algorithms, pitch and in 3D images by the reconstruction intervals.

Suffice to say that the detector size, pitch, reconstruction interval, and reconstruction algorithms play a key role in the determination of longitudinal resolution. The z-axis spatial resolution ranged from 1 to 10 mm in conventional (nonhelical) and in helical single-row detector CT (SDCT). In MDCT scanners with submillimeter detector size, the resolution in longitudinal direction is improved significantly and is approaching that of axial resolution

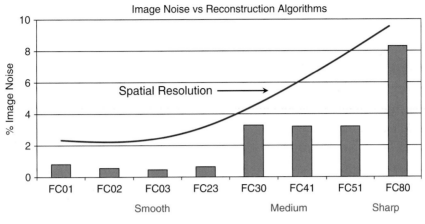

Figure 5.27. CT image noise (standard deviation of CT numbers within a region of interest) is affected by the type of reconstruction algorithms selected for image reconstruction. Image noise increases sharply with sharp reconstruction algorithms that yield high spatial resolution. Trade-offs between image noise and spatial resolution are achieved based on the desired CT image quality. With increased computing capability, the scan raw data sets often are reconstructed with various reconstruction algorithms to provide clinicians image sets of both high spatial resolution and low image noise.

striving to achieve isotropic resolution for CT images. The resolution is specified by measuring the slice-sensitivity profiles, which represents MDCT scanner response perpendicular to the scan plane. Full-width at half maximum (FWHM) and full-width at tenth maximum (FWTM) are measured on the slice sensitivity profiles as parameters to quantify the longitudinal

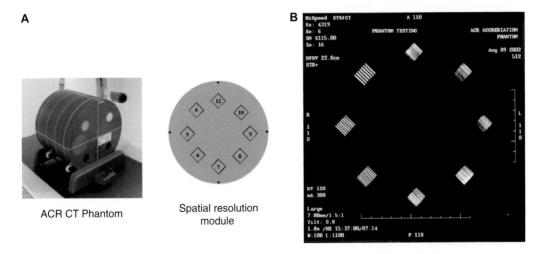

Figure 5.28. A: Spatial resolution module as part of the American College of Radiology CT accreditation phantom. The module consists of eight aluminum bar resolution patterns 4 to 10 and 12 lp/cm, embedded in background material with average CT number of approximately 90 HU. **B:** Spatial resolution image indicating resolvable rod size of up to 6 lp/cm (from McCollough CH and Brueswitz MR. The phantom portion of the American College of Radiology (ACR) Computed Tomography (CT) accreditation program. Med. Phys. 31 (9), September 2004: 2423–2442, with permission).

Table 5.3 Nominal spatial resolution and minimum object size resolvable by MDCT scanner in comparison with other imaging modalities

Imaging modality		Nominal spatial resolution, lp/mm	Minimum object size resolvable, mm
Nuclear medicine		0.1–0.072	5–7
PET-CT		0.1–0.07	5–7
MDCT	In-plane	0.5–2	1–0.25
	Longitudinal	0.7–1.5	0.7–0.3
Fluoroscopy		1	0.5
Radiography		1–10	0.5 to 0.05
Mammography	Digital	1–7	0.5 to 0.07
	Film-screen	5–20	0.1 to 0.05

Minimum resolvable size (mm) = 1/(2* nominal spatial resolution).

resolution. With 0.5–0.75 mm DAS channel width and double sampling, the best longitudinal resolution obtained currently is about 7–15 lp/cm (0.7–0.3 mm).

Overall, spatial resolution in axial or x–y plane has always been quite high and is of the order of 10–20 line-pairs per centimeter, whereas the longitudinal (z-axis) spatial resolution, which is influenced by the detector size, reconstruction slice, and other factors such as pitch, is around 7–15 lp/cm. Table 5.3 lists the nominal spatial resolution and minimum object size resolvable by MDCT scanner in comparison with other imaging modalities. The efforts towards obtaining isotropic resolution are leading further developments in MDCT technology.

Contrast Resolution. Low-contrast resolution is the capability of an imaging system to distinguish objects from its background. Low-contrast detectability (LCD) is an important indicator for any image system and high LCD means the system has high power to distinguish low-contrast objects from its background. LCD is the key discriminator for CT compared with other conventional radiographic systems and is often referred to as the sensitivity of the system. Because the slice thickness is smaller in CT (0.5 mm to 10 mm), the scatter is lower than the radiographic systems and therefore the low-contrast resolution is superior to radiographic imaging.

Contrast resolution is measured with phantoms containing low-contrast object with dif-

ferent sizes (Fig. 5.29). Contrast resolution performance of a scanner typically is defined as the smallest object that can be visualized at a constant image noise and dose and is dependent not only the size of the object but also its contrast (Fig. 5.29). In CT, low contrast detectability level is specified in terms of the percentage of linear attenuation coefficient. A 1% contrast means that the mean CT number of the object differs from its background by 10 HU.

There are number of factors that influence contrast resolution in CT, including x-ray photon flux (determined by tube current), slice thickness, patient size, detector sensitivity, reconstruction algorithm, and image display. The low-contrast detectability is significantly impacted by the noise in the background. If the background is very noisy, the LCD becomes poor. Because image noise in CT is affected by slice thickness, to improve LCD, CT images often are reconstructed into thick slices. The trade-off of thicker slices is poorer spatial resolution and the possibility of partial volume affect. With MDCT, there is no need to compromise spatial resolution to improve contrast resolution. With decreasing detector size and increasing computing capability, the mantra now is to acquire scan data with thinnest detector configuration available (provides high spatial resolution and three-dimensional images of isotropic resolution) and simultaneously reconstruct images by combining thin slices into thick slices to enhance contrast resolution.

A

B

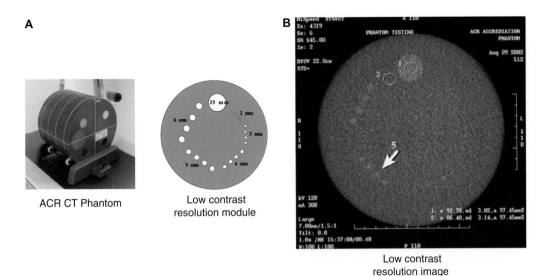

ACR CT Phantom

Low contrast
resolution module

Low contrast
resolution image

Figure 5.29. A: Low-contrast resolution module as part of the American College of Radiology CT accreditation phantom. The module consists of a series of cylinders of different diameters, all at 0.6% (6 HU) difference from background material with average CT number of approximately 90 HU. **B:** Low-contrast resolution image indicating resolvable rod size of up to 5 mm (from McCollough CH and Brueswitz MR. The phantom portion of the American College of Radiology (ACR) Computed Tomography (CT) accreditation program. Med. Phys. 31 (9), September 2004: 2423–2442, with permission).

Artifacts. Artifacts are misrepresentation of tissue structures seen in medical images. The imaging system may produce artificial structures that are deviation from the truth, resulting in artifacts. Compared with radiographic or fluoroscopic images, CT images are derived from a number of x-ray projections containing 1000 s of measurements, and these projections are back projected to reconstruct image. In this process, there is high probability for errors to occur as the result of inaccuracies in measurements, which can manifests as artifacts. Artifacts, if not properly identified and corrected, can lead to misdiagnosis.

Major types of artifacts that commonly are found in day-to-day clinical practice can be classified as *streaking artifacts, rings and band artifacts, partial volume artifacts, photon starvation artifacts, and patient-induced artifacts.*

Streaking artifacts are observed as intense, straight lines across the CT image and may appear as dark or bright (Fig. 5.30). These artifacts are caused by inconsistencies in individual measurements and are translated during the

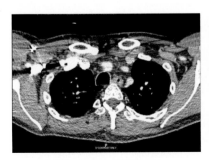

Thin images (0.75 mm)

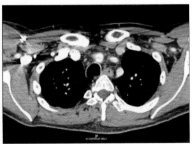

Thick images (3 mm)

Figure 5.30. CT image in the shoulder region shows streaking artifacts caused by photon starvation. Image quality compared to 0.75 mm CT images is improved by reconstructing thicker images (3 mm) images.

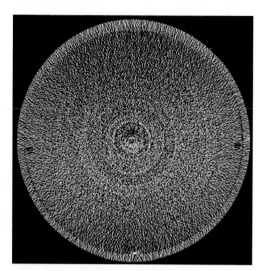

Figure 5.31. CT image of a water-filled phantom showing ring artifacts (from Barrett JF and Keat N. Artifacts in CT: Recognition and Avoidance. *RadioGraphics* 2004;24:1679–1691, with permission).

reconstruction process, yielding dark or bright lines across CT images. Streak artifacts are unlikely to cause misdiagnosis because they normally do not mimic any tissue structures; however, excessive streak artifacts can degrade image quality and can make images unreadable.

Ring or band artifacts appear as ring or band shapes superimposed on CT image. Ring artifacts can be either full or partial arcs. Full ring or band artifacts are easier to identify and are typical caused in third-generation type CT scanners (refer to Chapter 2 for details on generations) and are caused as the result of errors in single or multiple DAS channels in the detectors (Fig. 5.31). Partial ring or arcs are difficult to identify and can mimic tissue structures. Therefore, they can interfere in the diagnosis, as can the full rings, with a small radius appearing at the center of the CT image.

Partial volume artifacts occur when an object partially presents into the scanning plane. For example, scanning anatomy consisting of uniform density with partial intrusion from a high-density object results in inconsistencies between different views, causing shading artifacts to appear in the image. These artifacts are more common with thick slices (Fig. 5.32). Thick slices often are reconstructed to minimize image noise; however, the trade-off is the possibility of partial-volume artifacts. Partial-volume artifacts are best avoided by using thin slice acquisition, which is normally done with MDCT and is one of the reasons we are seeing fewer partial volume artifacts. Partial volume artifacts are a different problem from partial volume averaging, which yields an error in the average attenuation of the materials within the image voxel that can lead to inconsistency in quantification in CT.

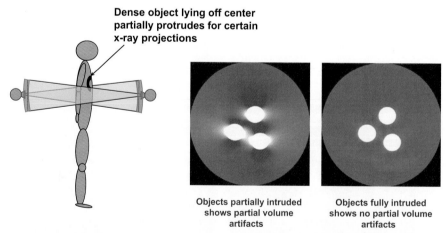

Dense object lying off center partially protrudes for certain x-ray projections

Objects partially intruded shows partial volume artifacts

Objects fully intruded shows no partial volume artifacts

Figure 5.32. Partial volume artifacts occur when a dense object lying off-center partially protrudes into path of x-ray beam in certain projections. Images obtained with dense objects intruded partially shows partial volume artifacts and objects intruded completely shows no partial volume artifacts (from Barrett JF and Keat N. Artifacts in CT: Recognition and Avoidance. *RadioGraphics* 2004;24:1679–1691, with permission).

Photon starvation artifacts are caused by a deficit in x-ray photons in certain areas. The applied technique may not be sufficient to penetrate the anatomy, especially while scanning obese patients, and can result in few x-ray photons reaching the detector, which in turn causes image noise. This artifact often is observed with increased image noise at the center of large patient scans. Photon starvation also can cause streak artifacts as the result of inconsistency in image formation. For example, scanning around shoulder region with uniform tube current can cause streak artifact (Fig. 5.30). There are methods to avoid photon starvation, such as adopting tube current modulation and adaptive filtration, which can provide sufficient x-ray photons while scanning around thicker object and yet keeping the radiation dose low.

Finally, the patient or the subject of interest that is scanned in CT causes artifacts. The *patient-induced artifacts* are the most common in CT. They are caused as the result of patient motion, beam-hardening effects, metal (inside and outside), and incomplete projections.

Patient motion artifacts are the most common type of artifacts found in CT. Patient motion can be either voluntary (respiratory, unrest as in case of pediatric patients) or involuntary (cardiac motion and other including bowel movement). Motion during data acquisition leads to inconsistency in projection data and leads to artifacts (Fig. 5.33). Although CT imaging is comparatively faster than other advanced imaging methods, patient motion results in a variety of artifacts. Patient-immobilizing devices can be used especially while scanning pediatric patients and, in rare cases, even sedations are performed.

However, the most widely used and effective method to reduce motion artifact is to instruct the patient to stay still and hold his or her breath during data acquisition. With faster and faster scans, it is now possible to complete most CT scan protocols with a single breath hold. In certain cases, patients are to be coached on how to breathe (shallow or symmetrical) instead of breath holding during CT scan (especially in PET-CT, since CT images are fused with PET images that are acquired with patient breathing normally. More discussion on PET-CT scans can be found in Chapter 9). Artifacts caused by car-

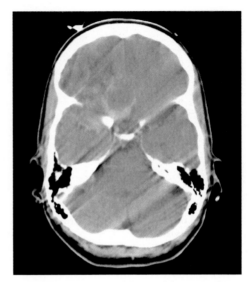

Figure 5.33. CT image of the head demonstrating motion artifacts (from Barrett JF and Keat N. Artifacts in CT: Recognition and Avoidance. *Radio-Graphics* 2004;24:1679–1691, with permission).

diac motion during cardiac CT scanning and the techniques adopted to minimize such artifacts are discussed in Chapter 6.

Beam-hardening artifacts appear as cupping or streaks or as dark zones between highly attenuating structures (bone). Beam hardening refers to the increase in the mean energy of the x-ray beam as it passes through the patient. Because the x-ray beam is composed of photons of varying energies and as x-rays passes through an object, it becomes "harder" (average energy become higher) as lower energy x-ray (soft x-rays) are absorbed more rapidly than higher energy x-rays. Beam hardening can induce variation in intensity as x-rays passes through objects, for example, in circular objects, the beam is harder passing through the center of the object compared with beam passing at the edges. The variation in x-ray beam energy yields cupping artifacts, which can mimic certain pathologies and lead to misdiagnosis (Fig. 5.34). Beam-hardening artifacts can be reduced by the use of adequate beam filtration, such as flat-filters and bow-tie filters, proper calibration correction, and beam-hardening correction software.

Metal artifacts are caused by the presence of metal objects inside patients such as metal prosthesis, pacemakers, clips, and stents or objects

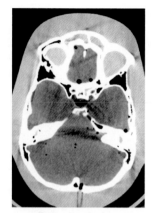 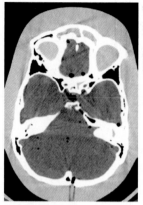

Beam hardening artifacts visible as dark bands   **Artifacts are less visible after beam hardening corrections**

Figure 5.34. Beam-hardening artifacts appear as dark bands between dense objects. Beam-hardening corrections applied during reconstruction diminish artifacts to a certain extent (from Barrett JF and Keat N. Artifacts in CT: Recognition and Avoidance. *RadioGraphics* 2004;24:1679–1691, with permission).

outside the patient such as jewelry, metal belts, and other effects wore by the patients. By simply instructing the patient to remove all external metal objects, such as jewelry, before scanning eliminates such artifacts. For in vivo metal objects such as dental prostheses, hip prostheses, and surgical clips, which cause streak artifacts as the result of beam-hardening, it is sometime possible to use partial scans to minimize the effects or to scan thin slices, which reduces some of the partial volume effects caused by metal artifacts. In addition, CT manufacturers have developed several metal artifact software correction algorithms that can be used to minimize the impact of metal artifacts. This becomes critical especially while scanning patients with hip prostheses. In the absence of beam hardening artifact correction algorithms, patients with hip

prostheses have limitations scanning abdomen and pelvis protocols (Fig. 5.35).

In addition, there are less common yet subtle artifacts caused by *scatter*, *artifacts* such as shading artifacts, *distortion artifacts*, and *aliasing* artifacts.

Scatter is one of the major causes of image degradation in x-ray images. X-rays in CT interacting with tissues undergo complete absorption (photoelectric effect) or scattering (Compton scattering) or simply pass through the object after attenuating to some extent, yielding required signal. Scattered x-rays reaching the detector results in lowering image contrast and also can yield shifts in CT number and lend to quantitative inaccuracies. Typically, scatter is removed by placing postpatient collimator. Typically in SDCT scanners, the scatter to primary ratio ranges less

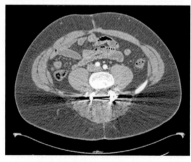 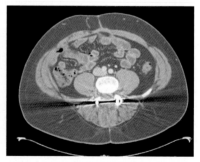

Thin images (0.75 mm)   Thick images (5 mm)

Figure 5.35. CT images of a patient with metal spine implants reconstructed with thin slice thickness (0.75 mm) and thick slice thickness (5 mm).

Table 5.4		Trade-offs that influence the choice of scanning parameters in both primary and secondary factors for MDCT

Parameters		Trade off
Scan parameters: primary factors		
Tube voltage (kVp)	High	Better penetration, less dose for given signal-to-noise in obese patients, especially in abdomen
	Low	Greater contrast (especially with iodinated contrast material), lower minimum dose, less dose for given signal-to-noise for children, slim patients, thin anatomical region
Tube current (mA)	High	Less noise, better contrast resolution, more patient dose
	Low	Less patient dose, more image noise, decreased detection of small low-contrast details
Scan time	Long	Long scan range, more motion artifacts, more contrast material required
	Short	Shorter scan range, improved temporal resolution, fewer artifacts, less contrast material required
Pitch	Large	Faster coverage or better z-axis resolution, less patient dose
	Small	Less spiral artifacts, increased patient dose
Scan length	Large	Large coverage, longer scan duration, greater patient dose
	Small	Short coverage, shorter scan duration, lower patient dose
Reconstruction parameters: secondary factors		
Field of view (FOV)	Large	Better overview, smoothing filter kernels are less disturbing
	Small	Greater maximum spatial resolution (requires HR filter kernels)
Slice thickness	Large	Less noise, better low resolution, more partial volume effects
	Small	Less partial volume effects, better z-axis resolution, more noise
Reconstruction interval (RI)	Large	Few images, but lesions may be missed
	Small	More images, better MPR/3D representations, more lesions detected
Reconstruction algorithm	Smooth	Less image noise and dose requirements, lower spatial resolution, better 3D images
	High	Substantially increased noise, greater spatial resolution
Geometric efficiency	High	Increased number of DAS channels
	Low	Fewer number of DAS channels
Spatial resolution	High	With thin detector configuration, sharp reconstruction algorithms
	Low	With thick slices, smooth reconstruction algorithms
Contrast resolution	High	With thick slices, with high mA
	Low	Thin slices, obese patients

than 5% whereas in MDCT with x-ray beam extending in the longitudinal direction, scatter to primary ratio can rise to as high as 50%.

Considerations are underway to adopt two-dimensional collimators in both axial and longitudinal planes to reduce scatter; however, introducing two-dimensional collimator similar to a grid can lead to the demand for increasing primary x-rays, resulting in a radiation dose to the patient. On the other hand, investigations are underway to adopt a complicated method of scatter corrections that, when applied appropriately, can even reduce overall radiation dose to the patient. In addition, energy-discriminating detectors may be a better solution to discriminate signals based on energy and because scatter is often composed of low-energy x-rays, energy-discriminating detectors can separate the scatter from primary x-rays, thereby providing opportunity to diminish scatter effects in CT images. Despite all the technological development in CT or in other imaging modalities, scatter continues to dodge eradication and cause image degradation. Finally, there are specific artifacts caused by inconsistencies in overall CT system design and x-ray detectors. These artifacts are rare and are often rectified and corrected by the CT manufacturer.

With MDCT scanners with wider beam width, the possibility of cone beam artifacts has become critical. Cone beam artifacts become increasingly worse with 16-row or greater MDCT scanners. Manufacturers are addressing many of these problems by using various forms of cone beam reconstruction techniques that are proprietary in nature.

In summary, artifacts originate from a range of sources and can degrade image quality, and certain cases can lead to misdiagnosis. Design features incorporated into modern MDCT scanner minimize many types of artifacts and some are partially corrected by scanner software. Still, many of the patient-related artifacts can be minimized with proper preparation of patients prior to scanning, positioning, optimum selection of scan parameters, and appropriate instruction (breath-holding) to patients.

Conclusions

There are number of scan parameters, both primary and secondary, that have an overall impact on CT image quality and radiation dose. The tradeoffs that influence the choice of scanning parameters are listed in the table (Table 5.4). Understanding each scan parameter—its role in the image formation, its interaction with other parameters, tradeoffs between image quality, and dose and patient comfort—helps to optimize CT protocols to achieve optimal image quality at minimal radiation dose.

6

Cardiac Imaging with MDCT

Coronary heart disease (CHD) represents the major cause of morbidity and mortality in Western populations. In 2005 alone, nearly 450,000 deaths were associated with CHD in the United States; that translates to nearly one of every five deaths. The economic burden on healthcare as the result of CHD is also enormous. Advances in multiple-row detector computed tomography (MDCT) technology have made it feasible to noninvasively image the heart and to evaluate CHD. Calcium scoring, CT angiography, and the assessment of ventricular function can be performed with MDCT. Coronary artery calcium scoring allows patients at intermediate risk for cardiovascular events to be risk stratified. Coronary arterial anatomy and both noncalcified and calcified plaques are visible in CT coronary angiography. Vessel wall pathology and luminal diameter are depicted, and secondary myocardial changes also may be seen.

The prospect of imaging the heart and coronary arteries with the use of CT has been anticipated since its development more than three decades ago. The lack of speed and poor spatial and temporal resolution of previous generations of CT scanners prevented the meaningful evaluation of the coronary arteries and cardiac function. Most early assessments of the coronary arteries with CT were performed with electron beam computed tomography (EBCT), which was developed in the early 1980s. EBCT has been used mostly for the noninvasive evaluation of coronary artery calcium, but other applications, including assessment of coronary artery stenosis, have been reported in limited cases.

Recent advances in CT technologies, especially MDCT, have dramatically changed the approach to noninvasive imaging of cardiac disease. With submillimeter spatial resolution (less than 0.75 mm), improved temporal resolution (80–200 ms), and electrocardiograph (ECG)-gated or triggered mode of acquisition, the current generation of CT scanners (16–320-multiple-row detectors) make cardiac imaging possible and have the potential to accurately characterize the coronary tree.

The objectives of this chapter are to describe the fundamentals of cardiac imaging physics with MDCT. In this work, the factors affecting temporal and spatial resolution are discussed along with scan acquisition and reconstruction methods, pitch, geometric efficiency, reconstruction algorithms, reconstruction interval, and radiation dose.

Key Issues of Cardiac Imaging with MDCT

The primary challenge required to image a rapidly beating heart is for the imaging modality to provide high temporal resolution. It is necessary to freeze the heart motion to image coronary arteries located close to heart muscles because these muscles show rapid movement during the cardiac cycle. Because the most quiescent part of the heart cycle is the diastolic phase, imaging is best if performed during this phase. Hence, it is required to monitor the heart cycle during data acquisition. The subject's ECG is recorded during scanning because the image acquisition and reconstruction are synchronized with the heart motion. Also, the imaging modality should provide high spatial resolution to resolve very fine structures, such as proximal coronary segments (i.e., right coronary ascending [RCA], left anterior descending [LAD] arteries) that run in all directions around the heart. These requirements impose greater demand on MDCT technology. One of the primary goals of the rapid development of CT technology has been to achieve these demands to make cardiac CT imaging a clinical reality.

Understanding the Physics of Cardiac Imaging

To better demonstrate and understand the necessity for high temporal resolution in cardiac imaging, Figure 6.1 shows how the length (in time) of the diastolic phase changes with heart rates. The least amount of cardiac motion is observed during the diastolic phase; however, the diastolic phase shortens with increasing heart rate. With rapid heart rates, the diastolic

phase narrows to such an extent that the temporal resolution needed to image such subjects is less than 100 ms. Desired temporal resolution for motion free cardiac imaging is 250 ms for heart rates up to 70 beats per minutes (bpm) and up to 150 ms for heart rates greater than 100 bpm. Ideally, motion-free imaging for all phases requires temporal resolution to be around 50 ms. The gold standard to compare temporal resolution obtained with MDCT is that of fluoroscopy, wherein the heart motion is frozen during dynamic imaging to a few milliseconds (1–10 ms). Therefore, the demand for high temporal resolution implies decreased scan time required to obtain data needed for image reconstruction and is usually expressed in milliseconds.

The demand is high for high spatial resolution that enables the visualization of various coronary segments (such as the RCA, LAD, and circumflex) that run in all directions around the heart with decreasing diameter. These coronary segments range from a few millimeters in diameter (at the apex of the aorta) to a few submillimeters in diameter as they traverse away from the aorta in all directions. The need to image such small coronary segments requires small voxels and is paramount to cardiac imaging with MDCT. Spatial resolution generally is expressed in line-pairs per centimeter or millimeter (lp/cm or lp/mm). Like temporal resolution, the gold standard for comparing spatial resolution is to that of the resolution obtained during fluoroscopy. However, one of the major goals of MDCT technology development has been to obtain similar spatial resolution in all directions, also expressed as isotropic spatial resolution.

In addition, a sufficient contrast-to-noise (CNR) ratio is required to resolve small and low-contrast structures such as plaques. In CT, low-contrast resolution typically is excellent. However, it can degrade with the increasing number of CT detectors in the z-direction yielding increased scattered radiation that can reach detectors in the z-direction. It is important to achieve adequate low-contrast resolution with minimum radiation exposure. The need to keep radiation dose as low as reasonably possible is essential for any imaging modality utilizing ionizing radiation. Overall, cardiac imaging is a

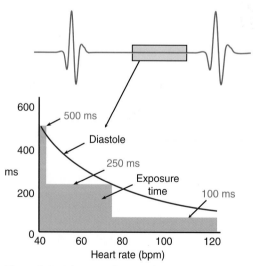

Figure 6.1. Schematic drawing showing the range of diastolic regions for varying heart rates. As noted, the desired temporal resolution for cardiac CT imaging is approximately 250 ms for average heart rates of less than 70 bpm and, for greater heart rates, the desired temporal resolution is approximately 100 ms.

very demanding application for MDCT. Temporal, spatial, and contrast resolution must all be optimized with emphasis on minimizing radiation exposure during cardiac CT imaging.

Temporal Resolution

There are a number of factors that influence the temporal resolution achieved on MDCT scanners. Among them the key factors are the gantry rotation time, acquisition mode, type of image reconstruction, and pitch.

Gantry Rotation Time. Gantry rotation time is defined as the amount of time required to complete one full rotation (360 degrees) of the x-ray tube/detector around the subject. Advances in technology have considerably decreased the gantry rotation time to as low as 330–370 ms (with a target of even lower than 300 ms). The optimal temporal resolution during cardiac imaging is limited by the gantry rotation time. The faster the gantry rotation, the greater the temporal resolution achieved. However, with increasing gantry rotation speed, there is also an increase in the stresses on the gantry structure, because the rapid movement of heavy mechanical components inside the CT gantry results in greater G-forces, making it harder to achieve a further reduction in gantry rotation time. In fact, even a small incremental gain in the gantry rotation time requires great effort in the engineering design. In the past, the minimum rotation time was as high as 2 s, and in the past few years, gantry rotation time has decreased steadily to less than 400 ms. As discussed in the previous section and in Figure 6.1, because the currently available gantry rotation time is not in the desired range for obtaining reasonable temporal resolution, various methods have been developed to compensate, such as different types of scan acquisitions or image reconstructions to further improve temporal resolution.

Acquisition Mode. For imaging the rapidly moving heart, projection data must be acquired as fast as possible to freeze the heart motion. This is achieved in MDCT either by prospective ECG triggering or by retrospective ECG gating.

Prospective Electrocardiogram Triggering. This is similar to the conventional CT *step-and-shoot* method. The patient's cardiac functions are monitored through ECG signals continuously during the scan. The CT technologist sets up the subject with ECG monitors and starts the scan. Instructions are built into the protocol to start the x-rays at a desired distance from the R-R-peak, for example at 60% or 70% of R-R interval. The scanner, in congruence with the patient's ECG pulse, starts the scan at the preset point in the R-R internal period, as shown in Figure 6.2. The projection data are acquired for only part of the complete gantry rotation (i.e., a partial scan). The minimum amount of projection data required to construct a complete CT image is 180 degrees plus the fan angle of the CT detectors in the axial plane. Hence, the scan acquisition time depends on the gantry rotation time. The best temporal resolution that can be achieved in the partial scan mode of acquisition is slightly greater than half of the gantry rotation time. Once the desired data are acquired, the table is translated to the next bed position and after suitable and steady heart rate is achieved, the scanner acquires more projections. This cycle repeats until the entire scan length is covered typically 12–15 cm (depending on the size of the heart).

With MDCT, the increasing number of detectors in the z-direction allows a larger volume of the heart to be covered per gantry rotation. For example, when using a MDCT scanner capable of obtaining 16 axial slices (16 rows of detectors with 16 data acquisition system (DAS) channels in the z-direction) with each detector having a width of 0.625 mm, one can scan a 10-mm (16 × 0.625 mm) length per gantry rotation. Similarly, with 64-slice MDCT scanner (64 row of detectors with 64 DAS channels) and each detector 0.625 mm wide, one can scan about 40 mm per gantry rotation. Typically the cardiac region ranges from 120 to 150 mm, which can be covered in three to four gantry rotations on a 64-row MDCT scanners. This has a major advantage in terms of the decreased time required for breath holding to minimize motion artifacts (critical when scanning sick patients).

One of the advantages of the prospective triggering approach is reduced radiation exposure, because the projection data is acquired for a

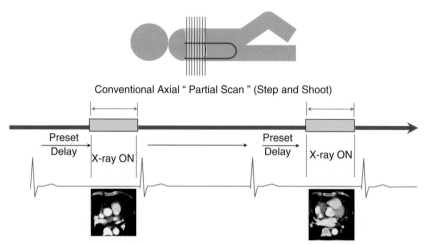

Conventional Axial " Partial Scan " (Step and Shoot)

Figure 6.2. During prospective ECG triggered scan mode, the patient ECG is continuously monitored but the x-rays are turned *'ON'* at predetermined R-R intervals to acquire sufficient scan data for image reconstruction. The table is then moved to the next location for further data acquisition. These types of scans are always sequential and not helical and results in lower patient dose because x-rays are *ON* for a limited period. Calcium scoring scans are typically performed in this scan mode.

short time periods and not throughout the heart cycle. Temporal resolution with this type of acquisition can range from 200 to 250 ms. Prospective triggering is the mode of data acquisition used for calcium scoring studies, since calcium-scoring analysis is typically performed in axial scan mode. The scan technique such as tube current (mA) for a calcium-scoring protocol can be quite low yielding low radiation dose, since calcium has a high CT number and is easily visible even with a noisier background. Also, each data set is obtained during the most optimal ECG signal to reduce motion artifacts.

Retrospective Gating. Retrospective gating is the main choice of data acquisition in cardiac coronary artery imaging with MDCT. In this mode, the subject's ECG signals are monitored continuously and the CT scan is acquired simultaneously in helical mode, as shown in Figure 6.3. Both the scan projection data and the ECG signals are recorded. The information about the subject's heart cycle is then used during image reconstruction, which is done retrospectively, hence it is called retrospective gating. The image reconstruction is performed either with data corresponding to partial scan data or with segmented reconstruction.

In segmented reconstruction, data from different parts of the heart cycle are chosen such that the sum of the segments equates to the minimal partial scan data required for image reconstruction. This results in further improvements in temporal resolution. Temporal resolution with this type of acquisition can range from 80 to 250 ms.

The disadvantage of retrospective gating mode of acquisition is the increased radiation dose, because the data are acquired throughout the heart cycle, even though partial data are actually used in the final image reconstruction. Also, because this scan is performed helically, the tissue overlap specified by the pitch factor is quite low, indicating excessive tissue overlap during scanning, which also increases radiation dose to the patients. The need for low pitch values or excessive overlap is determined by the need to have minimal data gaps in the scan projection data required for image reconstruction. The need for low pitch values is discussed in detail in the section on pitch.

Advantages and Trade-offs of Electrocardiogram Gating Versus Triggering. ECG gated retrospectively provides continuous coverage and better spatial resolution in the patient's

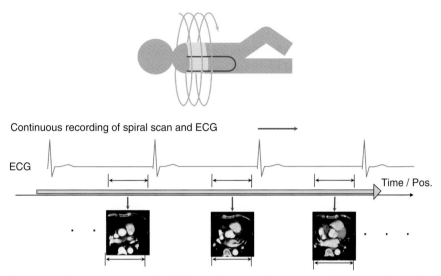

Continuous recording of spiral scan and ECG

ECG

Time / Pos.

Figure 6.3. During a retrospective ECG-gated scan mode, the patient ECG is continuously monitored and the patient table moves through the gantry. The x-rays are *ON* continuously and the scan data are collected throughout the heart cycle. Retrospectively, projection data from select points between R-R interval are selected for image reconstruction. Radiation dose is greater in these types of scan mode compared with prospective triggering method.

longitudinal direction because images can be reconstructed with arbitrary, overlapping slice increments. Instead, ECG-triggered sequential scanning usually is restricted to scanning non-overlapping adjacent slices with only small overlap. The scan time to cover the heart volume is directly proportional to the table increment.

Retrospective gating is less sensitive to heart rate changes during the scan. The ECG signal can be retrospectively analyzed and extrasystolic beats can be eliminated for reconstruction. With prospective triggering, the estimation of next R-R interval may be wrong when heart rate changes are prevalent (e.g., arrhythmia) and may result in data acquisition at inconsistent heart phases. Retrospective gating provides faster volume coverage than prospective triggering because scan data are acquired continuously and images can be reconstructed in every cardiac cycle. ECG-gated acquisition allows for imaging in a complete cardiac cycle using the same data set, thus providing cardiac function information. ECG triggering acquisition targets only one specific phase of the cardiac cycle and requires additional contrast agent to cover more phases of the cardiac cycle.

One of the major trade-offs of retrospective ECG gating is that data are acquired at small pitch values (0.2–0.4) and continuous x-ray exposure. Thus, ECG-gated acquisition requires greater patient dose than prospective triggering method for similar signal-to-noise ratios. All data acquired during ECG gating acquisition can be used for image reconstruction in different cardiac phases. However, if only one dedicated cardiac phase (middle of diastolic phase) is used, then rest of the data is omitted. Because there are numerous benefits of ECG-gated acquisition, methods currently are being investigated to reduce radiation dose with this method. Cardiac specific filters, optimization of pitch, and several other factors are considered to lower dose during retrospective gating.

With wide-area detectors such as 256- or 320-row MDCT scanners (0.5 mm of 256- or 320-row detectors with isoplane coverage of 12.8 cm or 16 cm), the entire heart can be covered with a wide-x-ray beam, resulting in the acquisition of data in a single heartbeat, and there is better opportunity to the lower radiation dose. This is discussed in chapter 10 on 256 row and 320 row MDCT scanners.

ECG Synchronization Methods. Except for 256- or 320-row MDCT scanners, where the entire cardiac data can be acquired in a single heartbeat, all other MDCT scanners require multiple heartbeats to cover the entire heart volume. In these scanners, with both types a of cardiac data acquisition, the ECG synchronization is critical. The starting points of data acquisition (prospective ECG triggering) or data selection for image reconstruction (retrospective ECG gating) have to be defined within each cardiac cycle during acquisition. These starting points are determined relative to the R-waves of the ECG signal by a phase parameter. The following ECG synchronization methods can be adopted (Fig. 6.4): relative delay and absolute delay forward or reverse.

Relative Delay. A preset time delay relative to the peak of the previous R-wave is used to determine the starting point of the ECG-triggered acquisition (as in prospective ECG triggering) or

the starting point of the reconstruction data interval (retrospective ECG gating). The time delay T_{del} is determined individually for each cardiac cycle as a given percentage of the R-R interval time T_{RR}. For example, the time delay may be 30–50% of the peak of the previous R-wave and can vary for each cardiac-cycle (Fig. 6.4A). For prospective triggering methods, the R-R interval time is estimated prospectively based on the previous R-R interval times.

Absolute Delay-Forward or Reverse. Fixed-delay time T_{del} after or before the onset of the R-wave (for example, 50% from the peak) will determine the starting point of the ECG-triggering acquisition or the start point of the reconstruction data interval. Absolute delay forward (Fig. 6.4B) is more practical than the absolute delay reverse method (Fig. 6.4C), because, in the latter method, the T_{RR} is estimated based on the previous R-R waves.

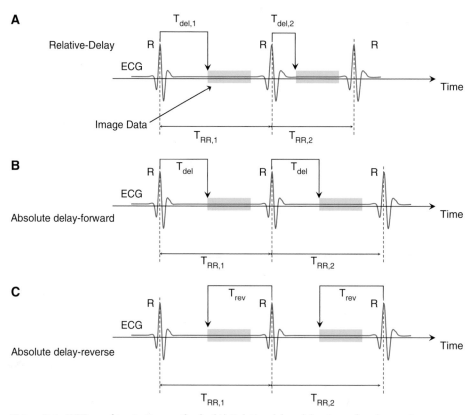

Figure 6.4. ECG synchronization methods: **(A)** Relative delay: delay time after the previous R-wave, determined as a percentage of the R-R interval; **(B)** absolute delay forward: a fixed interval after the previous R-wave; and **(C)** absolute delay reverse: a fixed interval of reverse time prior to the next R-wave.

Depending on the clinical practice, different approaches are in use. For motion-free imaging of cardiac anatomy in the diastolic phase with minimum cardiac motion, both are used most frequently. The least cardiac motion is present during the middle position of the R-R interval and, therefore, heart rate-dependent and patient-based optimization is critical to obtain best results. The challenge is during prospective triggering; often, the scanner has to wait before acquiring data. This can yield good motion free data sets, however, across many cardiac cycles.

On the other hand, in retrospective ECG gating, because the data are available through all phases of the cardiac cycle, it provides an opportunity of retrospective modification of synchronization of the ECG trace and data reconstruction. One can edit or omit certain R-R waves and select data snippets from various cardiac cycles for image reconstruction. Especially, in case of arrhythmia, certain R-R intervals can be deleted during the data reconstruction and still obtain motion free images.

For functional imaging with retrospective ECG gating, images are required to be reconstructed in phases of maximum or minimum filling of the ventricles (end-diastole or end-systole). End-diastolic reconstruction is feasible with absolute reverse method, whereas the absolute delay approach allows for most consistent reconstruction in end-systolic phase.

Reconstruction Method. Cardiac data acquired either by prospective ECG triggering or retrospective ECG gating is used in reconstructing images. High temporal resolution images are obtained by reconstructing either by partial scan reconstruction or by multiple-segment reconstruction.

Partial Scan Reconstruction. Among the methods of image reconstruction in cardiac CT, the most practical solution is the partial scan reconstruction. Partial scan reconstruction can be used for both prospective triggering and or retrospective gating acquisitions. The minimum amount of data required to reconstruct a CT image is at least 180 degrees plus the fan angle of data in the axial plane. This determines the

scan time to acquire projection data needed for partial scan reconstruction and also limits the temporal resolution that can be achieved from an acquisition. The CT detectors in the axial plane of acquisition extend in an arc that covers at least a 30- to 60-degree fan angle. Therefore, during partial scan reconstruction, the scan data needed for reconstruction are obtained by rotating the x-ray tube by 180 degrees plus the fan angle of the CT detector assembly as shown in Figure 6.5A. If the gantry rotation time is 500 ms, the time required to obtain the minimum scan data is slightly greater than half of the gantry rotation time. This means, for gantry rotation of 500 ms, the scan time for acquiring data for partial scan reconstruction is around 260–280 ms. These values represent the limit of temporal resolution that can be achieved through partial scan reconstruction.

To achieve further improvements in temporal resolution, the CT manufacturers are driving scanner gantry rotation time faster and faster. To date, the fastest commercially available gantry rotation time is around 300 ms. In such scanners, the partial scan reconstruction temporal resolution can be as high as 170–180 ms. At the same time, the G-force generated due to rapid gantry motion is growing exponentially and is reaching a limit for the existing technology. The demand for even higher temporal resolution has led to the development of dual-source CT and some are even considering developing multiple x-ray source CT scanners.

Multiple Segment Reconstruction. The primary limitation to achieving high temporal resolution with the partial scan approach is the gantry rotation time. To achieve even greater temporal resolution, multiple segment reconstruction was developed. The principle behind multiple segment reconstruction is that the scan projection data required to perform a partial scan reconstruction is selected from various sequential heart cycles instead of from a single heart cycle, as shown in Figure 6.5B. This is possible only with a retrospective gating technique and a regular heart rhythm. The CT projection data are acquired continuously throughout many sequential heart cycles. The multiple segment reconstruction method selects

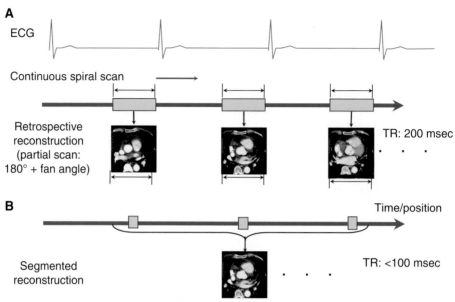

Figure 6.5. Differences between partial scan versus multiple segment reconstruction. **A:** As shown during partial scan reconstruction, sufficient data from prescribed time range between R-R intervals of one cardiac cycle is selected for reconstruction. **B:** In multiple segment reconstruction, sufficient data segments of same phase from multiple cardiac cycles are selected for image reconstruction. Greater temporal resolution can be achieved with this type of reconstruction.

a small portion of projection data from various heart cycles such that when all the projections are combined, they constitute sufficient data to perform partial scan reconstructions. For example, if one chooses to select half of the data set required for partial scan reconstruction from one heart cycle and the rest from another heart cycle, this results in temporal resolution that is about one-fourth of the gantry rotation time. This is done using projection data from two separate segments of the heartbeat cycle for image reconstruction. Further improvement in temporal resolution can be achieved by cleverly selecting projection data from three or four different heart cycles as shown in Figure 6.6, resulting in temporal resolution as low as 80 ms.

In general, with multiple segment reconstruction, the temporal resolution can range from a maximum of $T_R/2$ to a minimum of $T_R/2M$, where T_R is the gantry rotation time (seconds) and M is the number of segments in adjacent heartbeats from which projection data is used for image reconstruction. Usually, M ranges from 1 to 4.

$$TR_{max} = \frac{T_R}{2M}$$

$$T_R = 400\,\text{ms}, M = 1, \longrightarrow TR_{max} \geq \frac{T_R}{2} \geq 200\,\text{ms}$$

$$T_R = 400\,\text{ms}, M = 2, \longrightarrow TR_{max} \geq \frac{T_R}{4} \geq 100\,\text{ms}$$

$$T_R = 400\,\text{ms}, M = 3, \longrightarrow TR_{max} \geq \frac{T_R}{6} \geq 67\,\text{ms}$$

The advantage of multiple segment reconstruction is the possibility to achieve high temporal resolution. The disadvantage is that because projection data sets are obtained from different heartbeat cycles, a misregistration caused by rapid motion can result in the degradation of image spatial resolution. This method also allows selection of different packets of data for reconstructing an image for patients with irregular heart rates.

Overall, the temporal resolution of cardiac CT depends on the gantry rotation time. A gantry rotation time of 330–500 ms is possible with

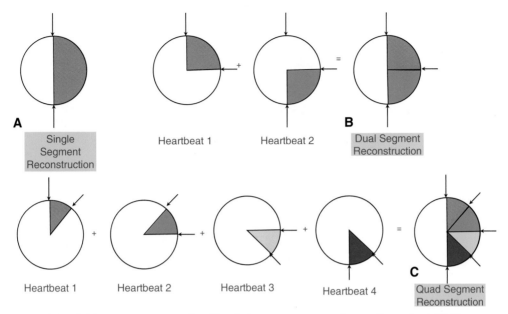

Figure 6.6. Multisegment reconstruction. The circles represent a complete cardiac cycle. **A:** Half-scan data are acquired during a single cardiac cycle in single-segment reconstructions. Half-scan data are acquired in two adjacent cycles in (**B**) dual-segment reconstructions and (**C**) in four adjacent cycles in quad-segment reconstructions. Temporal resolution can be improved to a quarter and an eighth of the gantry rotation time at dual and quad multisegment reconstruction, respectively, although spatial resolution may be degraded because of rapid cardiac motion.

16- to 64-row channel MDCT scanners. With such a rapid gantry rotation time, one can achieve a temporal resolution of 80–250 ms through multiple and partial segment reconstruction respectively. Temporal resolution improves with multiple segment reconstruction, as shown in Figure 6.7; however, the spatial resolution can degrade as the result of misregistration of motion artifacts because projection data sets are selected from different heartbeats.

With both the types of reconstruction, there is a demand for a significant amount of projection overlap during data acquisition, which is indicated by the pitch. Usually, the pitch ranges from 0.2 to 0.4 for cardiac CT protocols. This range is quite different from routine body CT protocols, which are typically performed with pitch values of 0.75–1.50.

Spatial Resolution. There are number of factors that influence the spatial resolution achieved with MDCT scanners. Among them are the detector sizes in the longitudinal direction, reconstruction interval, pitch, reconstruction algorithms, and patient motion.

Effect of Detector Size. The effect of detector size in z-direction or out of plane spatial resolution is very significant and has become one of the driving forces in the advancement of MDCT technology. Also, larger volume coverage in combination with larger number of thin images requires more detectors in the z-direction, which is the hallmark of technological advance in MDCT. On the other hand, scan plane or axial spatial resolution has been very high from the beginning and is dependent on the scan field of view (SFOV) and image reconstruction matrix. Axial pixel size is the ratio of SFOV to image matrix, for example for a conventional 512 × 512 matrix, the transverse pixel size for a 25 cm SFOV is 0.48 mm. On the other hand, the longitudinal or z-axis resolution mainly depends on the image thickness. The z-axis spatial resolution (image thickness) ranged from 1 to 10 mm in conventional (nonhelical) and in helical

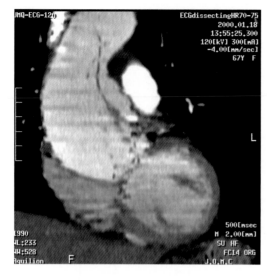 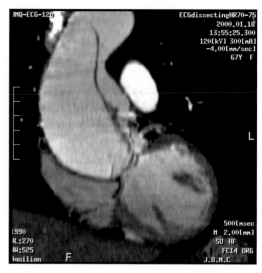

A Half-scan reconstruction
Temporal resolution: 250 msec

B Segmented reconstruction
Temporal resolution: ~105 msec

Figure 6.7. The effect of temporal resolution is demonstrated in the following images from the same patient. **A:** Partial scan reconstruction with temporal resolution of approximately 250 ms. **B:** Multiple-segment reconstruction (two segments) yielding a temporal resolution of approximately 105 ms. The stair-step artifacts are less visible and the image in the sagittal plane has smooth edge compared to partial scan reconstruction (from Toshiba Medical Systems, with permission).

single-row detector CT (SDCT). With MDCT, the z-axis detector size is further reduced to a submillimeter size. Initially, with the introduction of MDCT technology, the thinnest detector size was 0.5 mm, and there were only two such detectors. However, within a few years, the technology improved to provide 16 of these thin detectors, ranging from 0.625 to 0.5 mm. With 64-slice MDCT scanners, the detector array designs of 64 thin detectors (0.625 mm) result in z-axis coverage of up to 40 mm per gantry rotation. The increased spatial resolution with MDCT scanners is demonstrated in Figure 6.8. Cardiac CT can be comparable in delineating details of the coronary vessels to that of the cardiac images obtained with fluoroscopy.

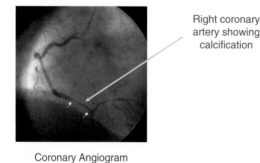

Right coronary
artery showing
calcification

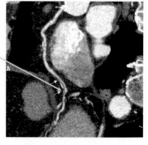

Coronary Angiogram

CT angiography

Figure 6.8. Right coronary artery showing calcification is observed on both cardiac CT angiographic and also on the fluoroscopically guided coronary angiographic images. The spatial resolution and delineation of details of CTA are comparable with coronary angiographic images (from Hoffmann MH. Pictorial essay. Noninvasive coronary imaging with MDCT in comparison to invasive conventional coronary angiography. *Am J Roentenol* 2004;182:601–608, with permission).

Reconstruction Interval. The reconstruction interval defines the degree of overlap between reconstructed axial images. It is independent of x-ray beam collimation or image thickness, and has no effect on scan time or patient exposure. The reason for decreased reconstruction interval (or increased overlap) is to improve z-axis resolution, especially for three-dimensional and multiple planar reconstruction (MPR) images. If the reader is making a diagnosis based on only axial images, reconstruction interval is not an issue. Frequently, however, physicians are also reading MPR and three-dimensional images; this is especially true for Cardiac CT. For example, in a single exam the same cardiac data set (acquired at 0.5 mm detector configuration) was reconstructed with three different values of reconstruction interval (Fig. 6.9A–C). Overlapping axial images results in a relatively large number of images but can also result in improved lesion visibly in MPR and 3D images without increasing the patient dose. For routine MPR and 3D applications, a 30% image overlap is generally sufficient (1-mm slice with a 0.7-mm reconstruction interval). For cardiac images, at least 50% overlap is desirable (0.5-mm slice thickness with 0.25-mm reconstruction interval).

It should be recognized that too much overlap results in a large number of images, increases reconstruction time, can result in longer interpretation periods, and can put undue strain on image handling overhead costs (image transfer, image display, image archive, etc) with no significant gain in image quality.

Overall, spatial resolution in axial or x–y plane has always been quite high and is of the order of 10–20 line-pairs per centimeter. The z-axis spatial resolution is influenced by the detector size, reconstruction thickness and other factors such as pitch, and is around 7–15 lp/cm. The efforts towards obtaining isotropic resolution are leading further developments in MDCT technology.

Pitch. The concept of pitch introduced with the advent of spiral CT and redefinition of the concept as applicable to both SDCT and MDCT is described in the previous chapter. The universal definition of pitch that is applicable to both SDCT and MDCT is the ratio of table increment per gantry rotation to the total x-ray beam width. Cardiac imaging demands low pitch values because higher pitch values result in data gaps, as shown in Figure 6.10, which are detrimental to image reconstruction. Also, low pitch values help to minimize motion artifacts, and certain reconstruction algorithms work best at certain pitch values, which are lower than 0.5 in cardiac imaging. Typical MDCT pitch factors used for cardiac imaging range from 0.2 to 0.4.

To illustrate these points, the pitch required during cardiac CT acquisition for a particular MDCT scanner that are generally affected by several parameters are shown in the following equations. For single segment reconstruction (partial scan acquisition), the pitch factor is influenced heavily by the subject's heart rate.

$$P \leq \left(\frac{N-1}{N} \right) \frac{T_{R}}{T_{RR} + T_{Q}}$$

Where N = number of active data acquisition channels (DAS);
T_{R} = Gantry rotation time (milliseconds);
T_{RR} = Time for single heart beat (milliseconds); and
T_{Q} = Partial scan rotation time (milliseconds)

For heart rates of 45–100 bpm (T_{RR} of 1333 to 600 ms, T_{R} of 500 ms, and T_{Q} of 250–360 ms), the required pitch factor ranges from 0.375 to 0.875. At higher pitch, there are substantial data gaps. As a result, most cardiac CT protocols require the infection of beta-blockers to lower the subject's heartbeat within the desirable range of <70 bpm. When the subject's heart rates are rapid and difficult to control, the diastolic ranges are smaller and therefore images are reconstructed with multiple segment reconstruction to improve temporal resolution. With multiple segment reconstruction, the numbers of segments used in the reconstruction further restricts the pitch factors.

$$P \leq \left(\frac{N+M-1}{NM} \right) \frac{T_{R}}{T_{RR}}$$

Where, N = number of active DAS channels;
M = Number of segments or subsequent heart cycles sampled;

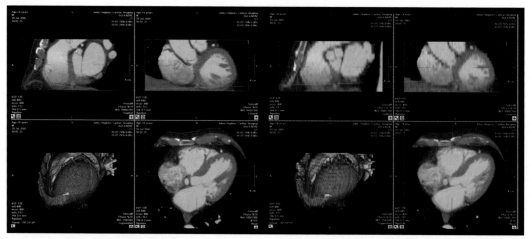

A SW 0.5 mm, RI 0.3 mm
301 images

B SW 0.5 mm, RI 5.0 mm
19 images

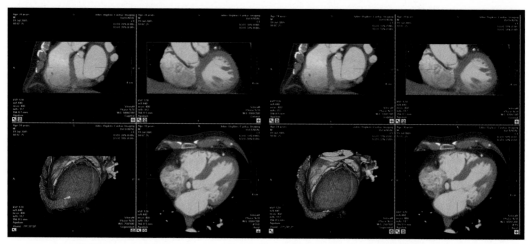

A SW 0.5 mm, RI 0.3 mm
301 images

C SW 0.5 mm, RI 0.5 mm
184 images

Figure 6.9. Impact of reconstruction interval on image quality: All three set of images shown are from the same data set reconstructed with 0.5-mm image thickness. However, the reconstruction intervals are different, which impacts on the number of reconstructed images and 3D image quality. **A:** Reconstruction interval is 0.3 mm, yielding 301 images and implying an 60% overlap. **B:** Reconstruction interval is 5 mm, yielding only 19 images resulting in staggered appearance in 3D images. **C:** Reconstruction interval is 0.5 mm yielding 184 images and image quality is similar to that of (**A**). Normally, a 50% overlap is sufficient for an optimum image quality for MPR and 3D images.

T_R = Gantry rotation time (milliseconds);
    and

T_{RR} = Time for single heart beat (milliseconds).

For a heart rate of 60 bpm, with a T_R of 400 ms, $N = 16$ and $M = 2$, the required pitch is ∼0.21 and, similarly, for $M = 3$, the required pitch is ∼0.15.

The pitch factor plays a significant role in both improving the temporal and spatial resolution but at the same time has a dramatic affect on the overall radiation dose delivered during a cardiac CT exam. Because radiation dose is inversely proportional to the pitch, the low pitch values characteristic of cardiac CT protocols substantially increase radiation dose

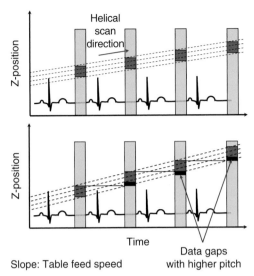

Figure 6.10. Graph demonstrating the necessity to scan at low pitch values during helical cardiac CT data acquisition. If the table feed becomes greater than the beam width, it results in data gap, which is detrimental for image reconstruction.

to patients undergoing cardiac imaging with MDCT.

In cardiac CT imaging, the need for high spatial and temporal resolution in turn requires the pitch values to be as low as 0.2–0.4. This results in a radiation beam overlap of nearly 80–60%, respectively, and an increase in radiation dose of up to a factor of five times compared with a pitch of one. Hence, proper choice and optimization of pitch factor is critical in cardiac imaging. In fact, the demand for reducing radiation dose and faster scan is driving the technology to introduce either even higher number of thin detectors in the z-direction (256 rows and 320 rows) or flat panel technology so that the entire cardiac area can be covered in a single gantry rotation without the necessity for tissue overlap (low pitch values).

Radiation Risk

Radiation dose in CT scanning is described in more details in chapter 7. Also, the radiation doses for various cardiac CT protocols are described in more detail along with other clinical protocols in chapter 7 radiation dose. However, a brief discussion on radiation dose as applied to cardiac imaging is presented here. The radiation dose delivered is highly dependent on the protocol used in cardiac CT. Among the most widely known protocols, such as calcium scoring studies, the effective dose, is relatively small, that is, 1–3 milli-Sieverts (mSv). However, for retrospective gating, which is used for coronary vessel stenosis assessment and CT angiography, effective doses of 8–22 mSv and greater have been reported. By comparison, the radiation dose of an uncomplicated diagnostic coronary angiography performed under fluoroscopic guidance ranges from 3 to 6 mSv and, for typical body CT protocols, ranges from 2 to 10 mSv (see Table 6.1). Across the board, radiation doses are higher with MDCT compared with the doses delivered using EBCT and fluoroscopically guided diagnostic coronary angiography similar procedures.

One approach to reduce the high dose associated with retrospective gating is called ECG dose modulation. It is directed at reducing the tube current during specific parts of the cardiac cycle, particularly during systole, where image quality is already degraded by motion artifacts and these portions of the cardiac cycle are not used in the image reconstruction. When dose modulation is implemented, a 10–40% dose reduction can be achieved; however, the savings must be evaluated for each specific CT protocol. Another method to lower dose is to perform most cardiac

Table 6.1 Typical effective doses for various cardiac and routine CT procedures

Procedures	Modality	Effective dose, mSv
Cardiac Procedure		
Ca Scoring	EBCT	1.0–1.3
Ca Scoring	MDCT	1.5–6.2[a]
Cardiac CT angiography	EBCT	1.5–2.0
Cardiac CT angiography	MDCT	6–7[a] to 25
Cardiac SPECT with Tc-99m or Tl-201	Nuclear medicine	6.0–15.0
Coronary angiography (diagnostic)	Fluoroscopy	2.1[a]–6.0
Chest x-ray	Radiography	0.1–0.2
Routine CT procedures		
Head CT	MDCT	1–2
Chest CT	MDCT	5–7
Abdomen and pelvis CT	MDCT	8–11

10 mSv = 1 rem.
[a] Hunold P, et al. Radiation exposure during cardiac CT: effective doses at multi-detector row CT and electron-beam CT. *Radiology* 2003;226:145–152.

CT protocols in prospective ECG triggering method. However, this approach has the risk of missing key data sets if the heartbeat varies rapidly during the scan. It is important that any steps taken to reduce radiation exposure should not jeopardize the image quality, because poor image quality may result in repeat scans, which would result in additional radiation doses to patients.

Artifacts

In cardiac imaging, because of the inherent nature of imaging a rapidly moving organ, there arises many unique artifacts, among them the most common artifacts are caused by cardiac pulsation. Figure 6.11 shows a disconnect in the lateral reconstructed image caused by pulsation. These types of artifacts are minimized by multiple-segment reconstruction or by scanning at even greater temporal resolution, that is, on the order of 50 ms. The second types of artifacts are the banding artifacts caused by increased heart rate during the scan. As shown in Figure 6.12, the heart rate varied from 51 bpm to 69 bpm during the scan and resulted in banding artifacts.

The other types of cardiac artifacts commonly observed are caused by incomplete breath holding on the part of the patient. These types of artifacts are not observed in axial images but are visible in coronal or sagittal views, as shown in Figure 6.13. When subjects with previous stents or coils in the coronary artery undergo CT imaging, we observe streak artifacts around these highly attenuating objects. Often these artifacts can dominate the artery region and obscure other structures. As shown in Figure 6.14, the metallic structures appear on axial images with no streak artifact but are very distinct and disturbing in coronal or sagittal planes. These types of artifacts are to some extent handled by special artifact reduction software developed by manufacturers. The blooming artifacts are caused primarily by the combination of very highly attenuating objects and the inherent limiting resolution of the scanner.

Future Directions in Cardiac Imaging

The demand for greater temporal and spatial resolution has led to the development of dual-source CT (DSCT) scanner and 256-row and 320-row MDCT scanners. A detailed discussion on DSCT and 256- and 320-row-MDCT scanners can be found in chapter 10 on advanced CT

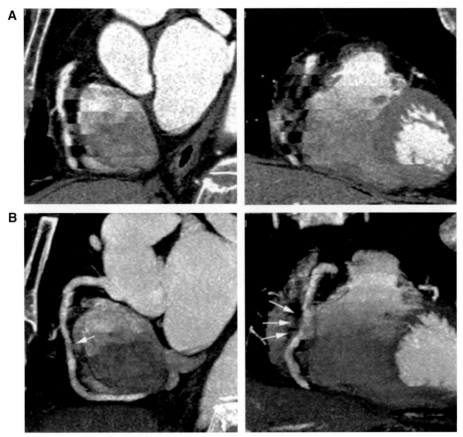

Figure 6.11. Cardiac pulsation artifacts due to rapid heartbeat are visible on **(A)** left anterior oblique and **(B)** anterior MPR images (From Nakanishi T. Pitfalls in 16–detector row CT of the coronary arteries. *RadioGraphics*, 2005;25:425–438, with permission).

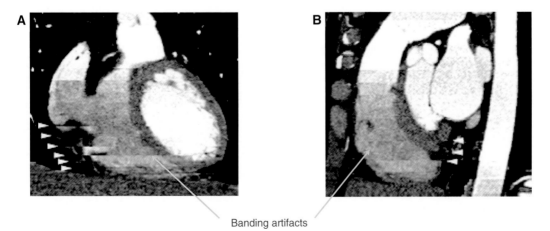

Banding artifacts

Figure 6.12. Banding artifacts due to increased heart rate form 51 to 69 bpm. Coronal **(A)** and sagittal **(B)** reformatted images of the heart obtained from CT data demonstrate banding artifacts (from Nakanishi T. Pitfalls in 16-detector row CT of the coronary arteries. *RadioGraphics* 2005;25:425–438, with permission).

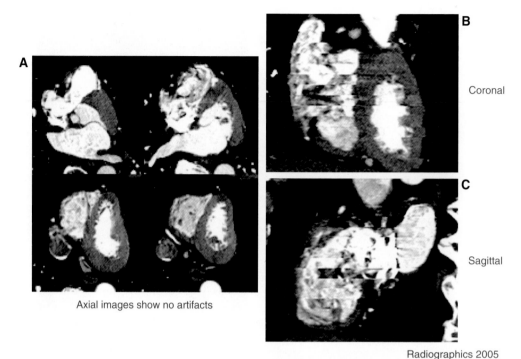

Radiographics 2005

Figure 6.13. A: Artifacts caused by incomplete breath holding. Axial images show no motion artifacts. Coronal (**B**) and Sagittal (**C**) reformatted images demonstrate banding artifacts (from Nakanishi T. Pitfalls in 16-detector row CT of the coronary arteries. *RadioGraphics* 2005;25:425–438, with permission).

scanning. A brief discussion on the two type of advanced MDCT scanner is given in chapter 10.

In DSCT, there are two x-ray tubes positioned 90 degrees apart, providing 64 axial slices for a complete gantry rotation, which yields further improvement in temporal resolution. As mentioned previously, the minimum data needed to reconstruct an image is 180 degrees plus the fan angle; therefore, with two tubes positioned at 90 degrees, it is sufficient to acquire data for one-quarter of gantry rotation and then coordinating the data from two sets of detectors to reconstruct the image. This can yield temporal resolution as low as one-fourth the gantry

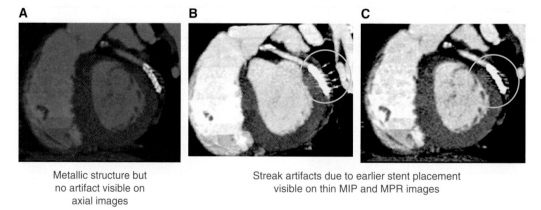

Figure 6.14. Streak artifacts visible in the presence of stent on (**A**) thin slab MIP, (**B**) MPR, and (**C**) thin slab MIP with wide window (from Nakanishi T. Pitfalls in 16-detector row CT of the coronary arteries. *RadioGraphics* 2005;25:425–438, with permission).

rotation speed. With scanner gantry rotation speeds at below 330 ms, the temporal resolution can be as low as 80 ms. With this scanner, the pitch factor may be increased for higher heart rates with a potential to reduce radiation dose.

Similarly, the demand for greater spatial resolution has led to the development of 256-row and 320-row MDCT scanner, which can cover the entire heart in one gantry rotation (12.8 cm and 16.0 cm beam width at isocenter, respectively). In the 320-row MDCT scanner, the 320 detectors in the longitudinal direction can cover an area of 16.0 cm per gantry rotation and therefore can eliminate the need for overlapping "pitch." In this type of scanner, it is possible to obtain complete data from one heart cycle, further diminishing the need for excessive tissue overlaps (low pitch values), therefore reducing radiation dose and also reducing motion artifacts. Ideally, the combination of 320-row detector assembly in the dual source CT would be phenomenal because that would not only give high temporal resolution but also high spatial resolution with minimal motion artifacts.

Conclusions

Cardiac imaging is a highly demanding application of MDCT and is possible only as the result of recent technological advances. Understanding the trade-offs between various scan parameters that affect image quality is paramount in optimizing protocols that can reduce patient dose. Benefits from an optimized cardiac CT imaging protocol can minimize the radiation risks associated with these cardiac scans. Cardiac CT has the potential to become a reliable tool for the noninvasive diagnosis and prevention of cardiac and coronary artery disease.

7

Radiation Dose

Computed tomography (CT) imaging is gaining widespread use not only in developed countries but worldwide. At the same time, concern about the radiation risk associated with CT scans is gaining attention. The importance of radiation dose from CT could be gauged by the attention given in public media and scientific literature on issue of radiation dose and the associated risks. The radiation dose levels in CT can exceed those from conventional radiography and fluoroscopy, and the use of CT continues to grow at a rapid pace, about 10% per year. In fact, according to one national survey, during 2007, approximately 67.8 million CT procedures were performed in hospitals and outpatient imaging facilities in the United States. Thus, the relative contribution of CT will continue to contribute significant part of the total collective dose delivered to the public from medical procedures involving ionizing radiation. According to recent National Council of Radiation Protection (NCRP) report, for United States in 2006, although CT examinations comprise only 17% of all the radiological examination (Fig. 7.1), CT contributes to nearly 49% of the effective dose of all radiological examinations.

The distribution of radiation in a CT scan is different from conventional x-ray or fluoroscopy. In the conventional radiography, the radiation dose is greatest as the x-ray enters the patient and least as it exits the patient. However, in CT, the x-ray tube rotates around the patient and, therefore, the surface dose is uniform and

maximum on the skin surface and decreases towards the center of the patient (Fig. 7.2). If the scanning volume is small, such as a head CT and or a pediatric CT, the surface dose is almost the same as the center dose. However, if the scan volume is large (in case of the abdomen region or in obese patients), the dose at the center of the scan region can be almost half ($\sim$50%) that of surface dose. For this reason, often there is increased image noise (grainy image) at the center of a large abdomen or in an obese patient, and proper adjustment of CT parameters is required to maintain optimal image quality.

Before discussing the radiation dose in CT, it is important to distinguish between the term *radiation exposure,* which relates to the amount of ionization created in air by the x-ray photons and the *absorbed dose,* which describesthe amount of radiation energy deposited in the patient's body as a result of exposure. The other key term associated with CT is the *effective dose,* which permits comparison of radiation with differing biological effects. Table 7.1 shows corresponding units and conversion factors. It is important to understand that *exposure* is a measured quantity outside the patient and the *absorbed dose* typically is calculated from the exposure and from estimation of how much energy is absorbed per body mass. Often the terms exposure and radiation dose are interchanged, which can cause some confusion when comparing doses among published literature.

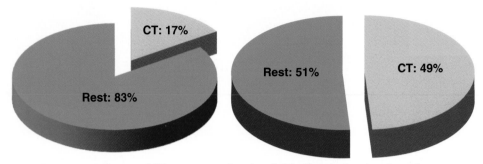

Figure 7.1. Percent contribution of CT examination (17%) and CT collective dose (49%) are shown in comparison with the overall medical radiological examinations in the United States for the year 2006 (From Mettler FA, et al. *Health Physics* 2008; 95:502–507).

CT Dose Descriptors

The fundamental radiation dose parameter in CT is the *CT dose index* (CTDI). There are many variants of dose parameters currently used in CT; among them, the following three, *volume CT dose index* (CTDI$_{vol}$), *dose length product* (DLP), and the effective dose (E), are important and have gained international acceptance to describe the CT dose. The effective dose parameter is useful in assessing and comparing the potential biological risk of a specific exam. Brief descriptions of each of these parameters are given below.

CT Dose Index. CTDI is the primary dose measurement concept in CT. Introduced in the 1970s, it represents the average absorbed dose, along the longitudinal axis, from a series of contiguous exposures. It is measured from one axial CT scan (one rotation of the x-ray tube around the CT gantry) and is calculated by dividing the total absorbed dose by the total x-ray beam width. CTDI usually is measured with thermoluminescent dosimeters (TLDs) and is labor intensive. It is more practical to measure with an ionization chamber of 100 mm length and the measurement is appropriately named CTDI$_{100}$.

The CTDI measurements are conducted with the use of standard polymethylmethacrylate (Plexiglas) phantoms of 16- or 32-cm diameter (Fig. 7.3A and B). The CTDI$_{100}$ measured in units of exposure (mR) is converted to absorbed dose (expressed in mGy). The typical dose distribution in CT as shown in Figure 7.2 is highest at the surface (patient skin) and decreases towards the center of the object. Therefore, for smaller anatomy (e.g., head CT), the skin dose and central dose are almost the same; however, for larger anatomy (e.g., abdominal CT), the central dose is nearly half of skin dose. This variation is accounted by taking the properly weighted average of the measured dose at the surface and at the center of the standard phantoms. The weighted CTDI (CTDI$_w$) is given as:

$$\text{CTDI}_W = 1/3 \ \text{CTDI}_{100,center} + 2/3 \ \text{CTDI}_{100,edge}$$

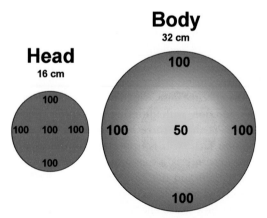

Figure 7.2. Typical dose distribution in CT examination. The radiation is uniform around the surface and is equal at both surface and at center for small objects such as head or pediatrics. The surface dose is nearly double that of central dose for large objects such as abdomen.

Typical values of CTDI are listed in Table 7.2 for different phantom diameters (head and body) and slice thicknesses or collimation, respectively. The CTDI values increases with decreasing slice thickness as the result of geometric efficiency (discussed in chapter 5).

Table 7.1	Radiation quantities and units		
Quantity	**Conventional unit**	**SI unit**	**Conversions**
Exposure[a]	Roentgen (R)	C/Kg	1 C/Kg = 3876 R (1R = 2.58 × 10^{-4} C/Kg)
Absorbed dose[b]	rad	Gray (Gy)	1 Gy = 100 rad
Effective dose[c]	rem	Sievert (Sv)	1 Sv = 100 rem

[a] Amount of charge created by ionizing radiation per unit volume in air.
[b] Energy deposited per unit mass of material by radiation.
[c] Permits comparisons of radiation with differing biological effects.

Although CTDI$_w$ is a useful indicator of scanner radiation output for a specific tube voltage (kVp), tube current (mA and mAs), and other factors, it represents the average absorbed dose in the axial plane only.

To represent dose for a specific CT protocol, which almost always involves a series of scans, it is essential to take into account any gaps or overlaps between the radiation dose profiles from consecutive rotations of the x-ray source. This is accomplished with use of a dose descriptor known as the *volume CTDI*.

$$CTDI_{vol} = (N \cdot T/I) \cdot CTDI_w \quad \text{applicable to sequential scans}$$

where N is the number of slices, T is the slice width, and I is the table increment between the consecutive slices.

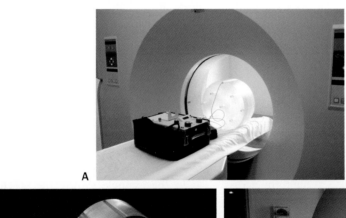

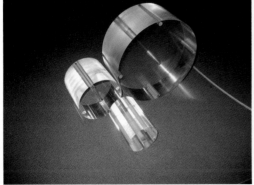

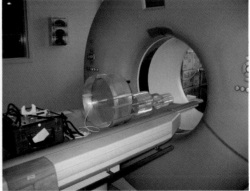

Figure 7.3. A: Typical setup for measuring CT dose index (CTDI$_{100}$). Shown is the standard abdomen phantom (32 cm in diameter) with ionization chamber (100 mm) positioned at the top surface of the phantom. **B:** Photograph of CT dosimetry phantoms, including body phantom (32 cm diameter), cranial phantom (16 cm diameter), and pediatric phantom (10 cm diameter).

Table 7.2   Typical CTDI values for different slice thicknesses measured for 16 cm (head) and 32 cm (body) CTDI phantoms at 120 kV on various Siemens CT scanners

Scanner	Scan mode, $N \times T$ mm[a]	Beam width, mm	Head CTDIw, mGy/100 mAs	Body CTDIw, mGy/100 mAs
Sensation 64	$32^{b} \times 0.6$	19.2	14.1	7.5
(64-MDCT)	20×1.2	24	12.6	6.7
Sensation 16	12×0.75	9	15.6	7.7
(16-MDCT)	16×0.75	12	11.9	7.2
	12×1.5	18	13.3	6.5
	16×1.5	24	9.9	6.5
Volume zoom	4×1	4	16.4	8.5
(4-MDCT)	4×2.5	10	13.7	6.9
	4×5	20	12.8	6.4
Somatom Plus	1×2	2	11.1	4.3
(SDCT)	1×5	5	11.2	6.4
	1×10	10	11.3	7.2

[a] N is the number of DAS channels, T is the DAS channel width.
[b] 32 physical detectors but each exposed twice to yield 64 slices.

However, for helical CT, because pitch is defined as the ratio of table travel per gantry rotation (I) to the total x-ray beam width ($N \times T$):

$$CTDI_{vol} = CTDI_{w}/pitch \quad \text{applicable to helical scans}$$

Volume CTDI. $CTDI_{vol}$ is the most accessible dose indicator because it is directly displayed on the MDCT scanner. It has gained global acceptance and provides some indication about the dose delivered to the patient. Because the method to derive $CTDI_{vol}$ is uniform across manufacturers and medical physicists, it can be used for direct comparison of the radiation dose from different scan parameter settings. However, one needs to understand that it does not provide an accurate dose to the patient but rather an index of dose from a particular scanner for a particular examination. $CTDI_{vol}$ should not be used to compare or assess individual risk.

$CTDI_{vol}$ remains same for a particular CT scan irrespective of how much anatomical region is scanned. However, the overall radiation dose delivered to the patient is different in both cases. This is accounted by the DLP.

Dose Length Product. DLP is indicator of the total radiation dose for an entire CT exam.

DLP represents the total dose for an entire CT exam, taking into account the total number of scans and the scan width. The definition of DLP is:

$$DLP \text{ (mGy-cm)} = CTDI_{vol} \text{ (mGy)} \cdot Scan \text{ Length (cm)}$$

It is expressed in mGy-cm.

For a select CT protocol, the $CTDI_{vol}$ remains same for all patients (because it is based on standard phantom and single measurement). However, DLP changes as the result of the difference in patient height.

In the example shown, the $CTDI_{vol}$ for a Chest CT are same in both situations (Fig. 7.4); however, the total radiation dose to the patient is greater in the second case because, in the second case, twice the anatomy is exposed to radiation. This difference is accounted by the DLP.

DLP increases with scan length for the same clinical protocol. These days, MDCT manufacturers are required to provide/display both $CTDI_{vol}$ and DLP at the end of each exam. A few scanners even allow users to save this information on separate file called a dose-report, which lists each series of CT scans along with key technical factors, $CTDI_{vol}$, and DLP for a CT exam.

As shown in Figure 7.5, some manufacturers display this information as a separate *dose report* for each patient. The information listed on the

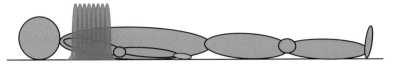

a. Chest CT: CTDIvol = 12 mGy, 16x0.75 mm, 8 rotations, **DLP = 115.2 mGy-cm**

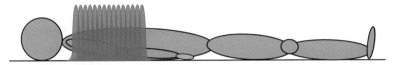

b. Chest CT: CTDIvol = 12 mGy, 16x0.75 mm, 16 rotations, **DLP = 230.4 mGy-cm**

Figure 7.4. Effect of scan length. Shown here are two scans (**A** and **B**) of a chest CT with different scan lengths. The CTDI$_{vol}$ is same for both cases; however, the DLP (dose length product) is double in the (**B**) because of the scan length.

dose report is based on standardized phantom measurements and this is quite helpful in assessing patient dose from a CT scan. In Figure 7.5, although both patients underwent a CT scan of the abdomen and pelvis, upon examining the dose report, it appears that subject (figure 7.5B) received an additional scan compared with subject 1. As the awareness of CT dose and risk

A

Total mAs 20002	Total DLP 2736						
	Scan	KV	mAs / ref.	CTDIvol	DLP	TI	cSL
Patient Position H-SP							
Topogram	1	120				7.8	0.6
ARTERIAL	2	120	450	32.31	1053	0.33	0.6
VENOUS	3	120	450	32.24	1683	0.33	0.6

B

Total mAs 28164	Total DLP 3873						
	Scan	KV	mAs / ref.	CTDIvol	DLP	TI	cSL
Patient Position H-SP							
Topogram	1	120				7.8	0.6
ARTERIAL	2	120	534	38.34	1212	0.5	0.6
VENOUS	3	120	530	38.02	1437	0.5	0.6
DELAY	4	120	500	35.96	1224	0.5	0.6

C

Total mAs 43773	Total DLP 5167						
	Scan	KV	mAs / ref.	CTDIvol	DLP	TI	cSL
Patient Position H-SP							
Topogram	1	120				7.8	0.6
ABDOMEN	2	120	400	28.74	1013	0.33	0.6
TestBolus	3	120	45	61.14	61	0.5	10.0
DS_CorCTA	27D	120	420	102.44	2761	0.08	0.6
AORTA	28	120	357	25.52	1332	0.33	0.6

Figure 7.5. Sample of CT dose reports. **A:** Dose report of a CT scan of the abdomen and pelvis with and without contrast. **B:** Dose report for a CT scan of the abdomen and pelvis that includes scan with, without contrast, and a delayed scan. **C:** Details of the CT angiography that includes bolus tracking and dual-source CT scans. The advantage of CT dose reports provides additional information such as list of all the CT scans performed within a CT examination.

grows, the utilization of dose reports will become key in assessing patient dose.

Although DLP represents most closely the radiation dose received by an individual patient, still $CTDI_{vol}$ is more useful in comparing radiation dose among various clinical protocols because it is not affected by the height of the patient (e.g., for a chest CT, with similar technical factors, the DLP is greater for a taller person than a shorter person).

For conventional (nonspiral) scanning, the scan length is simply the sum of all the slice collimations (e.g., 25 × 1 mm for 25 cm high-resolution CT). However, for spiral (helical) scanning, although one can use the difference between the table positions of the first and the last slice, the startup (ramping up of the helical scan) and stopping of the helical scan still results in additional partial rotations at the beginning and at the end and varies among MDCT manufacturers. The additional scan may be needed for image interpolations in the helical scans and is often called the *over-ranging* scan. This can contribute additional dose to the patient and if the scan length is small, the extra scans can become a bigger part of the overall dose to the patient. MDCT manufacturers have begun to pay attention to these extra helical scans by providing some sort of adaptive shielding that will block the radiation during these extra scans and expose only the desired anatomy.

Before ending the discussion on DLP, a similar dose descriptor can be found in fluoroscopy, where the dose parameter, called the dose-area-product ($mGy\text{-}cm^2$), is commonly used to assess risk to the patient undergoing prolonged interventional fluoroscopy. Knowing DLP alone is not sufficient because the final goal is to assess radiation risk to a patient undergoing CT scan. From DLP, one can estimate the *effective dose using* various methods.

Effective Dose. The effective dose is a dose parameter that reflects the risk of a nonuniform exposure in terms of a whole-body exposure. It is a concept used to "normalize partial body irradiations relative to whole body irradiations to enable comparisons of risk" (International Commission on Radiological Protection [ICRP 60], 1991). Because it is important to recognize that

the potential biological effects caused by radiation depend not only on the amount of radiation to the tissue or organ but also on the sensitivity of the tissue or organ, a radiation dose of 50 mGy to pelvis and 50 mGy to an extremity do not have the same biological effects as the result of variation in radiation sensitivity to different tissues or organs involved. *Effective dose*, or E, is the dose descriptor that reflects this difference and is expressed in units of milli-Sieverts (mSv).

The calculation of effective dose requires knowledge of the dose to specific sensitive organs within the body, which are typically obtained from Monte Carlo modeling of absorbed organ doses within mathematical anthropomorphic phantoms. Effective dose can be compared with the effective dose from other x-ray imaging modalities such as radiography or fluoroscopy or from other sources of ionizing radiation, such as that from background radiation level (e.g., radon, cosmic radiation, etc).

The concept of effective dose was originally designed for the protection of occupationally exposed individuals from radiation. It reflects radiation detriment averaged over sex and age, and its application has limitations when applied to medical procedures. However, it does provide a way to compare the biological effects of radiation between diagnostic exams of different types. When a patient asks, "What is the dose from a CT scan?" he or she is not expecting answers in terms of absorbed dose in mGy or so. In fact, the patient is indirectly asking "what is the risk from the CT exam?" Therefore, characterizing radiation dose in terms of effective dose provides a convenient way to communicate with patients and compare risks from other procedures or background.

Various computer programs are available that compute effective dose for a wide range of scanner types and organ systems. These programs can calculate the dose for individual organs, which is then appropriately weighted with the use of the organ-weighting factors from ICRP 60 to sum up and calculate effective dose E. Because the mathematical modeling done to compute organ doses is based on a standard adult (70 kg), effective dose estimation can underestimate the risk for children and thin patients and can overestimate the risk for obese patients.

Although effective dose calculations require specific knowledge about individual scanner characteristics, tissue-weighting factors for various organs, etc, a reasonable estimate of effective dose, independent of scanner type, can be achieved using the following relationship:

$$\text{Effective Dose} = k \cdot DLP$$

where, k is a weighting factor ($mSv \times mGy^{-1} \times cm^{-1}$), which depends only upon body regions (Table 7.3). The values of effective dose predicted by DLP and the values of effective does estimated using more sophisticated and elaborate calculations methods are remarkably consistent, with a maximum deviation from the mean of approximately 10–30%. Therefore, for routine purposes, the use of conversion factors for standard CT protocols has gained widespread acceptance. Table 7.4 provides a list of typical effective dose values for common CT exams. The annual level of natural background radiation in the United States is provided, which is a convenient way to compare patient doses. This allows an easier way to put CT doses into perspective and better understand the radiation exposure in a familiar context.

Effective dose, however, does not tell the complete story with regard to the potential effects of ionizing radiation. Specific organs and tissues are known to be more radiosensitive than others. Although this is reflected in effective dose, the absolute doses to specific organs or tissues also are important to consider, such

Table 7.4	Typical effective dose values for several common CT exams	
Examination		**Effective dose, mSv**
Head CT		1–2
Chest CT		5–7
Abdomen CT		5–7
Pelvic CT		3–4
Abdomen and pelvic CT		8–11
Calcium scoring		1–5
Cardiac CT angiography (helical)		10–20
PET-CT (whole body scans)		
CT portion	~10 mSv	20–25
PET portion (25 mCi FDG)	~15 mSv	

as in the case of fetal exposures, breast dose, and others. Typical dose values for critical organs are given in Table 7.5 for a few standard CT examinations to provide a perspective on the orders of magnitude to be expected. Along with the critical organ dose, effective dose is listed, which is the sum of all the organ doses weighted by the radiation sensitivity factors according to ICRP 60. Table 7.6a, b is a list of effective doses along with ranges of effective dose found on literature for CT and non-CT exams.

It is important to remember that the value of effective dose, E, whether computed by the use of elaborate methods or by simple conversion factors, is only an estimate. The many assumptions used in the calculation process are not accurate for any given patient. The $CTDI_{vol}$ calculated is based on the measurements performed on standard circular tissue equivalent phantoms. Therefore, one should remember that the uncertainty associated with the effective dose estimations could vary as much as 40% in certain cases.

In general, the biological effects of radiation are grouped into stochastic and deterministic risks. Stochastic effects are probabilistic in nature and typically effects 10–30 years from the time of exposure (long-term effects). Examples include radiation-induced cancers, mutations, etc. Deterministic effects, on the other hand,

Table 7.3	Standard conversion factors (k) for head, neck, chest, abdomen, and pelvis that are used for estimating effective dose (E, mSv) from DLP (mGy-cm) values[a]

Region of body	**k ($mSv \times mGy^{-1} \times cm^{-1}$)**
Head	0.0021
Neck	0.0059
Chest	0.014
Abdomen	0.015
Pelvis	0.015

[a] American Association of Physicists in Medicine, The Measurement, Reporting and Management of Radiation Dose in CT, Report No. 96, 2008.

Table 7.5	Typical effective doses for most common CT exams computed with simulation program (IMPACT dose calculator) and using standard conversion factors (Siemens Sensation 64)			
Anatomical region	**Head**	**Chest**	**Abdomen**	**Pelvis**
Scan length, cm	20	30	30	20
Slice thickness, mm	20×0.6	$64^a \times 0.6$	$64^a \times 0.6$	$64^a \times 0.6$
Voltage, kVp	120	120	120	120
Tube current $\times$ rotation time, mAs	400	200	250	250
$CTDI_w$, mGy	46.0	14.9	18.0	18.0
DLP, mGy – cm	920	420	540	360
Critical organ	Thyroid	Lung	Stomach	Colon
Organ dose, mGy	9	18	17	12
Effective dose, mSv	1.9	6.4	7.8	5.7
Conversion factor, mSv. mGy^{-1}. cm^{-1}	0.0021	0.014	0.015	0.015
Effective dose, mSv	1.9	6.0	8.1	5.4

[a] 32-row detector system capable of yielding 64 slices per x-ray gantry rotation.

exhibit a threshold dose below which the effects are not visible and above which the effects increases linearly with dose and are visible within in days to weeks. Examples include skin erythema, epilation, cataracts, even death.

Unlike interventional fluoroscopy, where deterministic effects are important, the stochastic risks are of great interest in CT. With advanced applications such as CT perfusion and CT fluoroscopy, the deterministic effects may also become important in CT. According to

BIER VII report, the risk of radiation-induced cancer (stochastic effect) is 5% per Sievert (Sv) (1 Sv = 1000 mSv). This means that there can be five additional radiation-induced cancers if all 10,000 people were exposed to 0.01 Sievert or 10 mSv. Although the risk is expressed uniformly across the age and sex, the risk varies with age and sex, as shown in Figure 7.6. Children are at two to three times greater risk than the general population for the same radiation dose because of a greater sensitivity to radiation.

Table 7.6a.	Representative effective dose (mSv) and ranges reported in literature for various CT procedures[a]	
Type of CT examination	**Effective dose, mSv**	**Range in literature, mSv**
Head	2	0.9–4.0
Neck	3	
Chest	7	4.0–18.0
Chest for pulmonary embolism	15	13–40
Abdomen	8	3.5–25
Pelvis	6	3.3–10
Liver, three-phase	15	5–25
Spine	6	1.5–10
Coronary angiogram	16	5.0–32
Calcium scoring	3	1.0–12
Virtual colonoscopy	10	4.0–13.2

[a] From Mettler FA, Huda W, Yoshizumi TT, Mahesh M. A Catalog of effective doses in radiology and nuclear medicine. *Radiology* 2008; 248:254–263, with permission.

Table 7.6b Representative effective dose (mSv) and ranges reported in literature for various diagnostic radiology procedures[a]		
Type of CT examination	**Effective dose, mSv**	**Range in literature, mSv**
Radiographic and fluoroscopy procedures		
Skull	0.1	0.03–0.22
Cervical spine	0.2	0.07–0.3
Thoracic spine	1.0	0.6–1.4
Lumbar spine	1.5	0.5–1.8
Chest, anteroposterior and lateral views	0.1	0.05–0.24
Mammography	0.4	0.10–0.60
Abdomen	0.7	0.04–1.1
Pelvis	0.6	0.2–1.2
Hip	0.7	0.18–2.71
Other extremities	0.001	0.0002–0.1
Dual-energy X-ray absorptiometry	0.001	0.001–0.035
Intravenous urogram	3.0	0.7–3.7
Upper gastrointestinal series	6.0	1.5–12
Small bowel series	5.0	3.0–7.8
Barium enema	8.0	2.0–18.0
Interventional procedures		
Head/neck angiogram	5.0	0.8–19.6
Coronary angiogram (diagnostic)	7.0	2.0–15.8

[a] From Mettler FA, Huda W, Yoshizumi TT, Mahesh M. A Catalog of effective doses in radiology and nuclear medicine. *Radiology* 2008; 248:254–263, with permission.

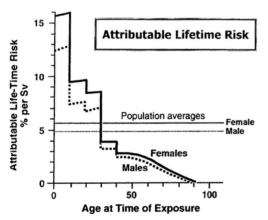

Figure 7.6. Attributable life-term risk versus age of time of exposure. Shown is the radiation risk (5% per Sievert) that is common for all ages but slightly different between male and female patients. In addition, the actual attributable lifetime risk is based on age and illustrates the point that the radiation risk is two to three times greater for pediatric population when compared with adult population. From ICRP Publication 60. Ann ICRP 1991; 21 (1–3), with permission.

Factors Affecting Radiation Dose and Image Quality

There are a number of factors that influence radiation dose during CT examinations, some greater than others. In the next section, the key factors that affect radiation dose are discussed.

Among the various factors, there are certain factors that are affected by the technical settings that are determined by the user and others are patient-related factors. Among the technical factors that affect radiation dose and image quality in CT are as follows.

Tube Current and Milli-Ampheres Second. Tube current (mA) in CT implies the amount of x-rays produced in the x-ray tube. The product of tube current and scan time (s) is milli-ampheres second (mAs). Both mA and mAs has linear relationship with respect to CT dose. The greater the mAs, greater is the patient dose. Also, the mAs impacts CT image noise. With all other technical factors kept same, if mAs is lowered, the radiation dose is lowered, and the CT image becomes grainy and noisy and vice-versa. As shown in Figure 7.7, three CT images of abdomen are simulated with of 48, 69, and at 184 mA, respectively, and the CTDI values shown under each image demonstrate the linear relationship between mA and radiation dose.

Certain CT manufacturers use the concept of *effective mAs*. Effective mAs is the ratio of mAs to pitch. To compensate for the decrease in image noise when pitch is increased, the mA is increased to maintain similar image noise. For example, with effective mAs of 200, with all other factors being the same (including scan time), there can be many combinations of mA and pitch. If the pitch is increased to 1.5, mA is increased to 300 mA to maintain same image noise. Similarly, if the pitch is decreased to 0.75, the mA is lowered to 150 mA.

Peak Tube Voltage. The peak tube voltage (kVp) is the peak potential difference between the anode and cathode, which accelerates the electrons toward anode to produce x-rays. The most common kVps used in CT scanners are 100–140

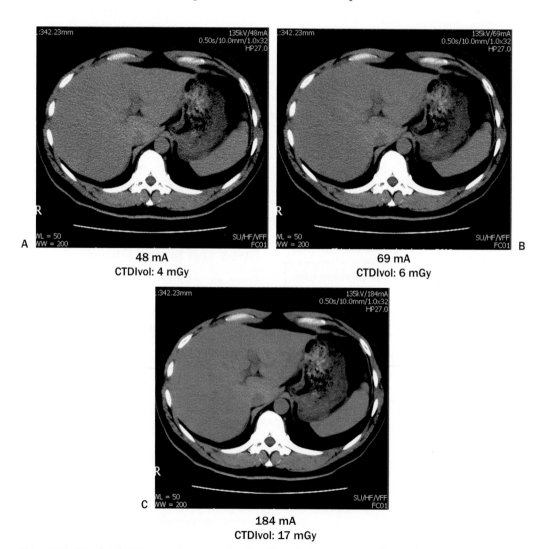

48 mA
CTDIvol: 4 mGy

69 mA
CTDIvol: 6 mGy

184 mA
CTDIvol: 17 mGy

Figure 7.7. Simulated CT images demonstrating the effect of tube current (mA) on radiation dose and image quality. Shown are three simulated images with similar scan parameters except with different tube current. The radiation dose increases linearly with increase in tube current.

kVp. kVp has a unique relationship with respect to radiation dose. The output of an x-ray tube is approximately proportional to kVp^2 and, therefore, if kVp is doubled, the radiation dose can increase by a factor of 4. kVp also affects the energy of the exiting x-rays, which influences the penetration capability of x-rays (Fig. 7.8). Therefore, increasing kVp increases the average energy of the x-rays, which can decrease subject contrast.

Tube voltages are not changed from patient to patient and are kept constant for a particular CT examination. Greater kVps such as 120–140 kVps normally are used for protocols that involve regions of greater attenuation, such as head, shoulder, or pelvis. Lower kVps, such as 80 and 100, are advantageous for scanning thin and pediatric patient. The effect of kVp on radiation dose and image noise is demonstrated in Figure 7.9A and B through simulated CT images of the head and abdomen respectively. For example, in Figure 7.9A, increasing kVp from 120 to 140 increases the $CTDI_w$ value from 12% to 29%.

Pitch. Pitch as defined in an earlier chapter is the ratio of table feed per gantry rotation to total x-ray beam width. Pitch plays unique impact on radiation dose during CT examination, as the radiation dose is inversely proportional to the pitch. Therefore, the greater pitch value, the lower the radiation dose and visa-versa. For abdominal and pelvic imaging, normally a P > 1 is sufficient. For certain protocols demanding high spatial resolution, P < 1 is used, resulting in greater patient dose. This is true especially with cardiac CT

scans, where the pitch is as low as 0.2–0.4 in certain cardiac CT angiography protocols. This translates to high patient dose in these scans. In Figure 7.10, simulated CT images of the abdomen are shown with varying pitch factors, which impacts both radiation dose and image quality.

Filters, Bow-Tie Filters, and Dose Profiles for Different-Sized Patients. Filters are absorbent materials inserted between the x-ray tube and the patient to absorb low energy x-rays (soft) and to harden the x-ray beam. The low-energy or soft x-rays contribute disproportionally to patient dose (especially to skin dose) and, therefore, it is desirable to harden the x-ray beam. As discussed earlier, filters increase the average energy of the x-ray beam. In CT, often the filter is shaped like a bow-tie to shape the x-ray beam to deliver a uniform intensity of x-rays across the scanning object, resulting in a more uniform dose distribution to the scanning region. Specific bow-tie filters are available for head, body, and cardiac and even for different-sized patients.

Beam-width. Beam-width implies the total x-ray beam exiting the x-ray tube and entering on the patient. It is defined at the isocenter of the CT scanner. In single-detector CT, the beam-width was called the slice-width. In MDCT, the beam width is the product of the number of data acquisition system channels and the thickness of each channels. Therefore, the beam width is 1 mm for detector configuration of 2 × 0.5 mm, 4 mm for 4 × 1 mm, 10 mm 4 × 2.5 mm, 20 mm for

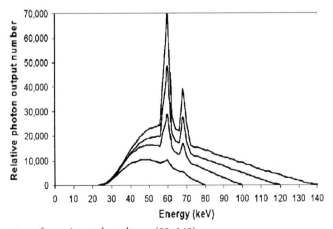

Figure 7.8. X-ray spectrum for various tube voltages (80–140).

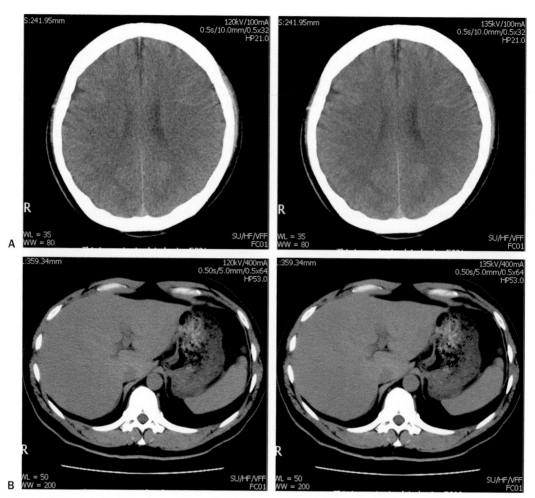

Figure 7.9. A: Simulated CT images demonstrating the effect of tube voltage (kVp) on radiation dose and image quality. Shown are two simulated images with similar scan parameters except with different tube voltage. An increase in 12% change in kVp leads to a nearly 29% greater radiation dose but only 14% decrease in image noise. **B:** Simulated CT images demonstrating the effect of tube voltage (kVp) on radiation dose and image quality. Shown are two simulated images with similar scan parameters except with different tube voltage. An increase in 12% change in kVp leads to a nearly 27% greater radiation dose and 25% decrease in image noise.

32×0.75 mm, and 40 mm for 64×0.625 mm, respectively (shown in Figure 7.11). Larger beam-width (160 mm with 320×0.5 mm) has unique advantage in covering large areas enabling wider anatomical coverage, thereby scanning entire organ such as heart in a single gantry rotation.

Variable mA Strategies. Variable mA strategies, also called *dose-modulation strategies,* imply modulating tube current while scanning across different anatomical region to reduce dose during the CT examination. Unlike automatic exposure control (AEC) in fluoroscopy,

CT does not have a true AEC control. Therefore, CT protocols often use the same mA for the entire study. With variable mA strategies, the tube current varies as the patient's thickness changes from the neck to shoulder to chest and abdomen. Various dose reduction strategies adopted by different CT manufacturers are discussed at length in the next chapter.

Repeats. With multiple CT scans, the radiation dose to patient increases. In certain protocols, CT examination may include multiple scans such as CT of the chest, with and without

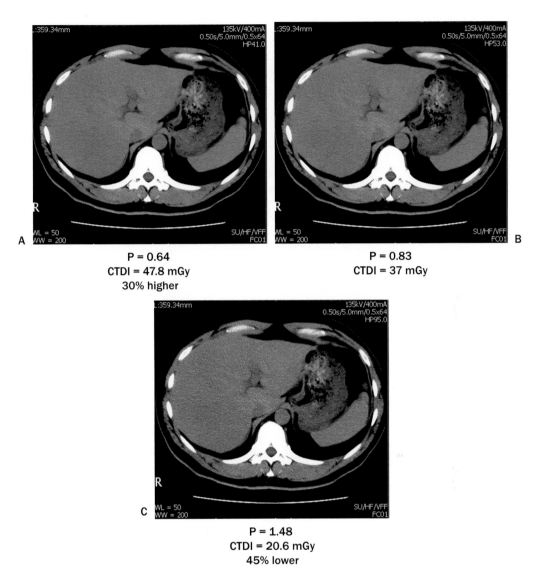

P = 0.64
CTDI = 47.8 mGy
30% higher

P = 0.83
CTDI = 37 mGy

P = 1.48
CTDI = 20.6 mGy
45% lower

Figure 7.10. Simulated CT images demonstrating the effect of pitch on radiation dose and image quality. Shown are three simulated images with similar scan parameters except with different pitch values. A pitch of 0.64 results in an increase of nearly a 30% greater radiation dose compared with a pitch of 0.83. Similarly a pitch of 1.48 leads to a decrease of a nearly 45% in radiation dose. Depending on the type of scan and image quality, often pitch greater than 1 is quite sufficient for routine imaging. The only protocols that demands very low pitch (0.2 to 0.4) are with retrospective cardiac CT angiography examination.

contrast, triphasic liver study involving three scans (Fig. 7.5: dose reports). At the outset, it appears that during a single visit to the CT suite, the patient may be scanned multiple times. In addition, patients often undergo multiple CT exams in a short period of time. How many of these scans are necessary and how many are inappropriate is a critical question with no single answer. Multiple CT scans are a concern for patients because of the radiation exposure. The radiation dose increases with each additional CT scan. The stochastic effects are the main biological effect of radiation that is a concern with CT scans. Although stochastic effects of radiation are not additive, each CT scan increases the probability of stochastic effects.

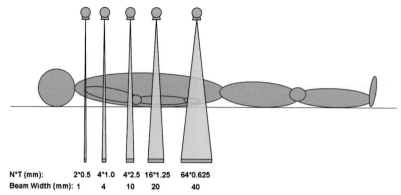

| N*T (mm): | 2*0.5 | 4*1.0 | 4*2.5 | 16*1.25 | 64*0.625 |
| Beam Width (mm): | 1 | 4 | 10 | 20 | 40 |

Figure 7.11. Schematic drawing the increase in x-ray beam width with each generation of MDCT scanners. The product of number of data channels and width of each data channel determines the total x-ray beam width defined at the isocenter of the CT gantry.

Dose efficiency in MDCT. Dose efficiency (also called geometric efficiency) is of particular concern with narrow beam collimation in CT protocols. In MDCT, it is required that roughly equal numbers of x-ray photons strike all active detectors in the z-direction. This requirement means that there is certain amount of *over-beaming* of the primary x-ray beam beyond the active detector surface that results in radiation dose penalty (Fig. 7.12). The proportion of radiation wasted relative to the overall width of the x-ray beam varies with the protocol used. If a CT scan is performed with few thin detectors configuration (e.g., 4 × 0.5 mm) the dose penalty is more compared with the same scan done at a thick detector configuration (for example 16 × 0.5 mm). The effect of dose efficiency is demonstrated in Figure 7.13, where normalized values of $CTDI_{vol}$ are shown among 4-, 16-, and 64-channel MDCT scanners from the same

manufacturer. The CTDIw shows significantly higher results for 4-channel scanner compared with the 16- and 64-channel scanners. Dose increases markedly with narrowing beams and fewer active detector elements but less so for wider beam and more detectors as the result of improved geometry efficiency.

Shields. Shielding the region adjacent to the primary area of CT scans has advantages in limiting radiation that exceeds the scan region (especially during helical CT scans). Shielding certain organs that are in the primary area of CT scan is drawing attention these days. Studies have shown a reduction in breast dose when bismuth shields are placed over the breast during CT scans of chest and heart. Placing shields on the breast during chest and cardiac CT may reduce some amount of incident x-rays to the breast at certain angles; however, there is the

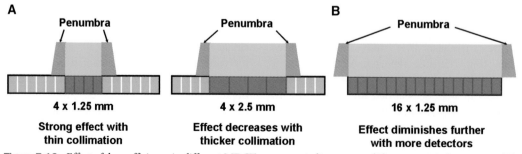

A

Penumbra

4 x 1.25 mm

**Strong effect with
thin collimation**

Penumbra

4 x 2.5 mm

**Effect decreases with
thicker collimation**

B

Penumbra

16 x 1.25 mm

**Effect diminishes further
with more detectors**

Figure 7.12. Effect of dose efficiency in different MDCT scanners: 4-slice scanner (**A**) versus a 16-slice scanner (**B**).

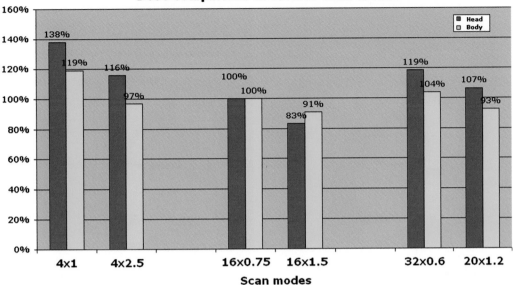

Figure 7.13. CTDI$_{vol}$ values (normalized to the 16-slice scanner values) for 4- (left), 16- (center), and 64- (right) slice MDCT scanner from the same manufacturer. The 4-slice acquisitions deliver greater dose index values than the 16- and 64-slice acquisitions owing to poor dose efficiency. Red bars indicate head CT dose, yellow bars indicate body CT dose.

possibility of image artifacts and diminished image quality beneath the shielded area. Overall, the use of patient shields has to be evaluated carefully, taking into consideration such as logistics of using the shields in a clinical environment (cost, time, and hygiene are key factors to be considered), the impact of shields when dose-modulation techniques are applied, and when to place the shields on patients (placing the breast shield after the scout scan has a greater impact when dose modulation is applied). No matter what types of shields are used, there will be a certain amount of internal scatter that cannot be avoided. On the other hand, optimizing the protocol by reducing mA for the entire protocol may have greater effect on radiation exposure to patient than certain patient shields.

The second type of shielding is related to personal shielding for those inside the CT scanner suite during a procedure such as CT biopsy or CT fluoroscopy. During CT fluoroscopy, the physician performing the procedure stands very close to the CT gantry, which cluds the area of greatest scatter radiation. Therefore, it is critical that anyone inside the CT suite use appropriate shields.

Reconstruction. Image reconstruction does not have any influence on the CT dose to the patient. With the increased computing capability these days, the scans on a patient are performed with one technique and later reconstructed with a variety of reconstruction algorithms, which basically implies that once the desired data are acquired, they can be reconstructed into multiple phases and multiple data sets with no direct impact on radiation dose (Fig. 7.14). Often, scans are performed with a thin detector configuration, such as 64 × 0.625 mm, so that the raw data enables the user to reconstruct CT images at very high resolution, key to 3D images, and also in thick slices to reduce image noise (Fig. 7.15). Also, with single raw-data sets, various reconstruction algorithms can be applied to obtain various image data sets.

The patient factors that influence total dose during CT are size of the patient, scan length, number of CT exams, genetic susceptibility, and also the age and sex of the patient.

Patient Size. The technical factors set for CT exam has to be changed based on the patient size.

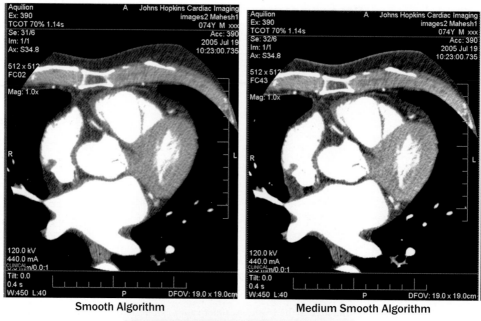

A   Smooth Algorithm   Medium Smooth Algorithm   **B**

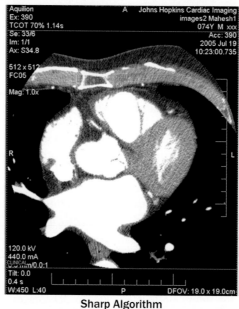

C   Sharp Algorithm

Figure 7.14. Effect of reconstruction algorithms on image quality. The advantage of high computing capability provides CT users an opportunity to reconstruct raw CT data with different reconstruction algorithms to demonstrate images with higher spatial resolution or lower image noise. The availability of various reconstruction algorithms allows CT users to reconstruct CT images depicting different image quality aspect without having to repeat the CT scan.

For larger patients, in order for x-rays to penetrate through large area, it becomes necessary to alter technical factors such as tube current and tube voltage. In such a patient, the displayed $CTDI_{vol}$ is not an accurate indicator of the dose to the patient.

Age. As discussed earlier, the risk associated with radiation is higher for younger patients, in fact the risk is two to three times greater for children undergoing CT for the same dose as that of adult.

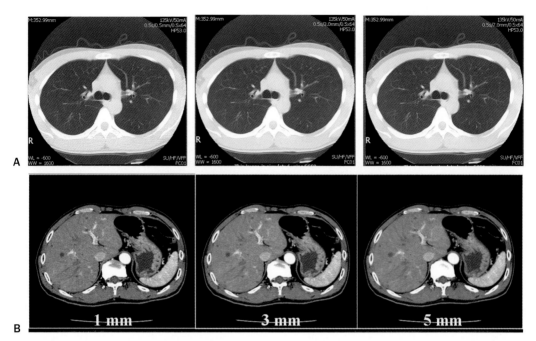

Figure 7.15. Effect of slice thickness on image quality demonstrated with chest CT images (**A**) and Abdominal CT images (**B**) reconstructed with different slice thickness. Thin images are sharper, yielding greater spatial resolution but also greater image noise. On the other hand, thicker slices provide images with lower image noise and reduced sharpness. With 16- and 64-slice MDCT scanners, it is often advantageous to acquire data with the thinnest-possible detector configuration and later reconstruct both thin (desired for three-dimensional images) and thick images (low image noise) providing both high spatial resolution images and low noise images.

Table 7.7	Effect of scan parameters on patient dose and image quality
Parameter	**Effect on patient dose**
Tube current	• Increases or linearly with mA value
Tube voltage	• No simple relationship between voltage and patient dose.
	• Influences penetration
Scan time	• Increases or linearly with scan time
Pitch	• Inversely proportional to dose
	• Lower pitch (<1) leads to higher dose
	• Higher pitch (>1) leads to lower dose
Thin slices	• Increases patient dose especially when lower slices are prescribed
	• For example: 4 × 0.5 mm dose penalty higher than 64 × 0.5 mm
Beam filtration	• Higher beam filtration is advantageous to block soft x-rays
Scan length	• Increases linearly with scan length
	• Lower dose due to shorter exposure time
Cardiac CT	
Prospective triggering CT angiography	• Lower dose because data acquired through partial portion of the ECG signal
	• Limited data set
Retrospective gated helical CT angiography	• Higher dose because data acquired throughout ECG signal, even though only partial data is used in image reconstruction

Sex. The radiation risks varies with sex; especially when certain critical organs such as breasts are in the field, the risks are greater in women compared with men. Certain CT protocols such as cardiac CTs yield greater radiation exposure to the breast in women. Care should be taken to optimize the dose when critical organs are in direct path of the primary x-rays.

Scan length. For any CT exam, the total dose is influenced by length of the scanned regions. Taller patients will have a greater DLP compared with shorter patients and therefore have greater effective dose values for the same CT examinations. DLP values should not be used as a dose indicator to compare doses among patients undergoing similar CT examinations.

Conclusions

For CT scans, the radiation doses typically are greater than the conventional radiography but are comparable with certain interventional fluoroscopic and nuclear medicine procedures. Even though the risk from CT is small, with the increasing use of CT, the associated radiation risks are not negligible. The amount of radiation required to do a CT scan has to be kept as low as reasonably achievable (i.e., ALARA). In Table 7.7, the effects of various CT scan parameters on radiation dose are given.

There are many factors both technical and patient related that affect radiation dose during CT examination. In the next chapter, various dose saving strategies developed by different MDCT manufacturers are described in details.

In summary:

(i) $CTDI_{vol}$ is the most accessible dose indicator readily available at the scanner allows direct comparison of radiation dose for different technical factors and for various CT manufacturers.

(ii) $CTDI_{vol}$ is not an accurate dose representation for any individual patient, but is rather an index of dose for a particular scanner and examination.

(iii) $CTDI_{vol}$ underestimates the average dose within the scan volume for children and slim patients and overestimates for obese patients. The displayed $CTDI_{vol}$ has to be corrected for children protocol.

(iv) DLP varies with patient's height.

(v) Effective dose (E) is not measured for each patient but is estimated based on standard circular size phantoms. The uncertainty in the effective dose estimation can vary as much as 40%.

(vi) Among the various factors that affect radiation dose, tube current, tube voltage and pitch plays a significant role.

8

Strategies to Reduce Radiation Dose in CT

Introduction

Recent technological advances have markedly enhanced the clinical applications of computed tomography (CT). There has been a remarkable increase in use of CT since its inception in the early 1970s, and the number of CT procedures performed in the United States has been growing about 10% annually since 2000. According to a recent National Council on Radiation Protection (NCRP) report, although the CT procedures accounts for only 17% of all medical x-ray procedures, it accounts to about 49% of the total radiation dose associated with medical imaging in the United States. Whereas the benefits of CT exceed the harmful effects of radiation exposure in patients, increasing radiation doses to the population have raised a compelling case for reduction of radiation exposure from CT. It is critical to examine or develop methods to reduce radiation dose without compromising image quality.

In the absence of true automatic exposure controls as found in other x-ray imaging modalities such as radiography and fluoroscopy, it is important how CT scanning is performed so as to adhere to ALARA principle (as low as reasonably achievable) and at the same time not compromising the CT image quality. In this regard, major CT manufacturers have developed various strategies to reduce radiation dose in their multidetector row CT (MDCT) scanners. These strategies can be broadly grouped either as hardware improvements or as software improvements, including image reconstruction algorithms, tube current modulations, and so forth. In this chapter, strategies to reduce radiation dose as applicable to their respective MDCT scanners is presented by each major MDCT manufacturer and is arranged according to the alphabetical order of their names.

GE Healthcare MDCT Scanner Strategies to Reduce Radiation Dose
■ Thomas Toth and Jiang Hsieh, PhD

In this section, we describe some of the dose management methods available on GE Healthcare CT Scanners. These methods are included in: (i) Hardware design and implementation; (ii) Software features to optimize image quality at reduced radiation levels; and (iii) System software for x-ray exposure control.

Hardware Design and Implementation

Suppression of Off-Focal Radiation. Dose reduction begins within the x-ray tube. Secondary electrons that bounce off the anode after their primary impact on the focal spot are

115

randomly attracted back to the anode causing off-focus radiation. Off-focus radiation increases patient dose and degrades image quality by creating artifacts near abrupt anatomic changes such as bone edges and by increasing image noise. GE Healthcare CT x-ray tubes include a specially designed backscattered electron suppression ring that captures secondary electrons to minimize this source of unwanted x-rays, reducing dose about 5% and minimizing artifacts.

X-Ray Beam Filtration. When appropriately matched to the patient, the x-ray beam quality and the shape of the beam intensity profile are effective way to optimize the dose efficiency using fundamental x-ray physics principles. The scan field of view (SFOV) selection by the user selects both the x-ray beam filtration that establishes beam quality and the bowtie filter that determines the shape of the x-ray beam intensity within the scan field. The name of the SFOV is associated with the filtration that would generally be most appropriate for the indicated patient anatomy. GE Healthcare MDCT scanners provide multiple bowtie filters and two levels of beam quality filtration. For heads and pediatric selections, the small or medium filter provides an x-ray field with a narrow shape and a softer beam quality that is optimized for anatomy up to 30 cm in diameter. The softer beam quality improves tissue contrast and the narrow x-ray field reduces surface dose for smaller patient anatomy that is appropriately positioned. For cardiac scanning, when the region of diagnostic interest is only the heart, the small and medium filters can provide a dose savings and image contrast improvement. The large bowtie filter has a wider x-ray intensity shape

with a harder beam quality. The large bowtie filter is optimized for larger anatomy. In larger anatomy, low energy (soft) x-rays are absorbed as patient dose and therefore do not reach the detector to contribute to the image. The large filter reduces the soft x-ray content to minimize this source of unwanted dose in large patients. The wider x-ray field shape of the large bowtie provides sufficient x-ray intensity to maintain image quality over the larger diameters while providing a dose reduction for the surface regions of the patient. Bowtie filters can reduce surface dose exposure up to 50% compared to an x-ray field of uniform intensity.

Z-Axis Geometric Efficiency—X-ray beam tracking and Focal Spot Size. A MDCT scanner requires a uniform x-ray field (umbra) to be positioned over the Z-axis extent of the detector to provide consistent image quality over all detector rows. The edge portion of the Z-axis profile that diminishes in x-ray intensity (penumbra) cannot be used for imaging and thus contributes to patient dose if not properly managed. The goal is to maintain this penumbra region as narrow as possible by appropriate selection of the focal spot and by using closed loop beam tracking collimation to minimize the overall x-ray beam width. The small focal spot is automatically selected for any exposure that does not require high tube power. The small focal spot reduces the penumbra region nearly in half. In addition, an active beam tracking system constantly monitors the position of the beam on the detector and repositions the collimator every few milliseconds to maintain the penumbra snugly against the edge of the detector (Fig. 8.1). Active beam tracking is needed since the position of the focal spot will

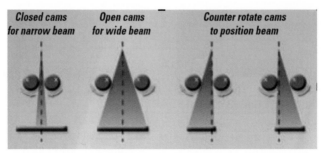

Figure 8.1. Interactive and continuous correction of the x-ray beam is performed with focal spot tracking to adjust the x-ray beam every few milliseconds to maintain narrow x-ray beam.

change due to thermal and mechanical factors. Without tracking, the source collimator would need to be opened much wider to maintain the detector within the wandering umbra as the focal spot moves. The source collimator on GE Healthcare MDCT scanners is a set of cams that are easily rotated to restrict the x-ray over the Z-axis active portion of the detector that is being used to collect the data for making images.

Shutter Mode Collimation. The GE Health-care source collimator is highly suited to block much of the helical over ranging radiation at the beginning and ending of a helical scan. Although efficient helical reconstruction algorithms are employed to minimize helical over ranging, some of the detector row data that extends beyond the image region is not needed for image reconstruction as the patient image region transitions into and out of detector z-axis x-ray field. GE Healthcare is currently developing a shutter mode that will dynamically rotate the cam collimator to block unneeded transition radiation from the unused portion of the detector.

Data Acquisition System. Large patients and low x-ray techniques in regions such as the pelvis or shoulders present a significant challenge for a CT data acquisition system (DAS). This is because x-ray signal levels are low compared to inherent electronic circuit noise. Under extreme low signal conditions, the electronic noise begins to dominate the data that can cause severe image degradation. The GE Healthcare DAS technology minimizes electronic noise by combining the following elements: (i) A *HiLight*™ or *Gemstone*™ scintillator material with a 99% x-ray detection efficiency and an intense light signal output characteristic. (ii) Backlit photodiodes that allow electrical interconnections without blocking any light and thereby devoting 100% of the sensitive area to capturing scintillator light even with very small detector pixels. (iii)Miniaturization of the electronic circuitry to minimize pickup of interfering signals and reduced electrical signal lead lengths to reduce undesired capacitance. The result is a compact and efficient DAS that does not add significant electronic noise even at very low photon flux levels.

Software Features to Optimize Image Quality

Adaptive Filtration. Image space smoothing filters as well as the selection of a soft reconstruction kernel can reduce image noise but such filters can also soften the edges of image features along with the noise. GE Healthcare has provided a class of filters that adapt in accordance with image characteristics within a local region of image voxels. These adaptive filters adjust their performance depending on voxel statistics. In voxel regions with characteristics indicative of the presence of a gradient (image feature), the filter can perform smoothing in the direction of the gradient and even slightly enhance the edge perpendicular to the gradient. An isotropic smoothing filter is applied only in voxel regions that statistically have a low probability of containing an image feature. This adaptive process can preserve or make anatomic features easier to distinguish within a reduced noise background and thereby allow improved image quality or the opportunity for reducing dose.

Another form of adaptive filtration is employed in projection space on the view data prior to image reconstruction. In large highly asymmetric patients, image noise can create a deep streaky artifact pattern. GE Healthcare scanners provide level dependent filtration to the view data prior to image reconstruction. This filtration is applied only to those views where it is needed at a level that is calibrated in accordance with the signal level of the view and its associated noise contamination. This projection space adaptive filtration is always in operation analyzing view data and functions only when needed without any user initiated settings.

(i) **Three dimensional neuro-adaptive filters** are sets of adaptive algorithms, specifically tailored for brain imaging, that perform volumetric image analysis to identify regions with and without anatomic structures and perform isotropic smoothing operations on the non-structure regions and edge preservation or sharpening on the structured regions. There are 3 levels of filtration (high medium and low) available for user selection in head protocols, resulting in up to a 30% noise reduction to improve image quality or to allow dose to be reduced for scanning.

(ii) **Adaptive filtration for ECG-gated cardiac imaging**-cardiac imaging is especially challenging and prone to higher image noise. This is due to the use of very short scan times with lower mAs or when the heart phase may vary unexpectedly causing increased image noise for the selected ECG mA modulation (discussed below). The increase in noise can be managed to some extent by using adaptive filters specifically designed for cardiac imaging. GE Healthcare currently provides three cardiac imaging adaptive filters designed to reduce noise and preserve edges specifically for the heart anatomy in cardiac imaging modes. The most aggressive filtration is designed to improve image quality and allow a reduction in dose especially when imaging obese patients. Dose reductions of 10% to 30% have been achieved using these adaptive filtration algorithms (Fig. 8.2).

Iterative Reconstruction Algorithms.
Iterative reconstruction (IR) is a class of reconstruction algorithm that generates cross-sectional images from measured projections of an object. The algorithm has been applied extensively in emission tomographic modalities such as single photon emission computed tomography (SPECT) and postron emission tomography (PET). In x-ray computed tomography, however, this method is not currently in use on medical scanners largely because of its significantly slower computational speed as compared to the filtered backprojection methods (FBP) are currently available on all commerical CT scanners.

Iterative Reconstruction. GE Healthcare is agressively researching *Model-based Iterative Reconstruction (MBIR)* algorithms. These algorithms have been shown in recent years to have the potential for drastic image noise reduction while improving spatial resolution and reducing image artifacts at the same time. Noise reduction in the reconstructed images can often be used to reduce x-ray radiation dose to the patient by lowering the CT scanning techniques. With the MBIR approach, the noise versus resolution tradeoff curve is significantly different from that of the traditional filtered backprojection (FBP) algorithm and allows a better visualization of the small objects without the signficant penalty of noise increase. The advantages of MBIR are the results of the algorithm's ability to accurately model the CT system.

In the conventional FBP approach, many simplified assumptions have to be made in order to make the mathematics manageable. For example, the physical sizes of the x-ray focal spot and the detector cell are assumed to be

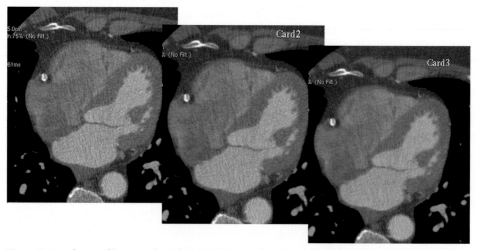

Figure 8.2. Adaptive filtration algorithm for ECG-gated cardiac images demonstrates reduction in noise and preservation of edges in cardiac region.

infinitely small; the shape of the reconstructed image voxel is ignored, and the measured signals are assumed to be perfect. These assumptions naturally lead to suboptimal image quality since they deviate from reality. MBIR, on the other hand, tries to model the optics of the CT system by taking into consideration the actual sizes and shapes of the focal spot, detector cells, and image voxels. In addition, noise properties of the entire CT system are properly modeled.

In studies to compare MBIR performance with FBP algorithms, MBIR demonstrated up to an 80% noise reduction as compared to a high-resolution FBP algorithm while still improving spatial resolution, in the axial plane (x-y plane) and in the longitudinal direction (z-axis). When MBIR is commercially available, it is expected to dramatically improve image quality and allow substantial dose reduction.

Adaptive Statistical Iterative Reconstruction Algorithms. Although MBIR is effective in improving spatial resolution and reducing noise in the reconstructed CT images, the computational complexity is high and the reconstruction speed can be too slow for routine clinical applications. A first step in the implementation of the MBIR algorithm into practical usage is *Adaptive Statistical Iterative Reconstruction (ASIR)*, introduced on GE Healthcare's most recent scanners. Instead of modeling the entire CT system, ASIR focuses only on the

modeling of the statistical properties of the imaging chain. As a result, the computational complexity of ASIR is significantly reduced which allows its routine clinical usage on special computer hardware. Phantom and clinical evaluation have shown up to 40% improvement in low-contrast detectability and up to 50% dose reduction while maintaining image quality (Fig. 8.3).

Color-Coding for Kids. GE Healthcare has adopted a color-coding scheme based on the *Broselow-Luten pediatric measuring system*. This system is used in many emergency rooms and other pediatric care facilities to reduce the likelihood of improper medication use and to ensure that correct size accessories are employed. In the *Broselow-Luten* system, nine color categories are assigned based on patient weight and length and each patient is fitted with the proper colored bracelet. The goal of the GE Healthcare *Color Coding for Kids* system in CT is to simplify the protocol selection process for pediatrics. The objective is to reduce the likelihood of errors when scanning protocols are selected without regard to patient size (weight and length), since this could result in using higher than needed dose levels. The scan protocol selection interface allows operators to use the same color codes to select the appropriate predefined protocol that provides the right amount of dose for the imaging task. This color scheme guides the operator to select protocols based on patient weight and

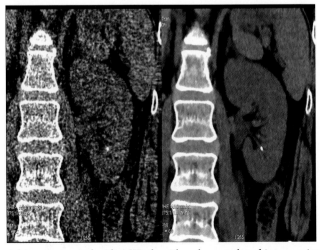

Figure 8.3. Image on right reconstructed with ASIR algorithm shows reduced image noise and improvement in low contrast detectability compared to image on left.

height information and thus reduces the chance of errors. Combined with a suitable choice of *noise index* or mAs selection for the imaging task, the use of *Color Coding for Kids* can result in considerable lower dose protocols and more consistent image quality across a wide range of pediatric patient sizes (Fig. 8.4). Modifications of this scheme have been implemented to take into account recent recommendations to adjust dose based on the diagnostic task and number of prior scans in addition to size and anatomic region.

Dose Recording and Display. GE Healthcare scanners provide a standard dose display on the console to show the CTDIvol, CTDI

phantom size and DLP for the selected scan settings. In addition, this same dose report information is available on a text page image. Current new GE Healthcare scanners also provide a DICOM structured dose report that allows dose information to be electronically recorded, transmitted and analyzed.

System Software for X-ray Exposure Control

AutomA. *Automatic exposure control (AEC) software for CT imaging, such as the GE Healthcare AutomA,* automatically determines the tube current as a function of patient size to maintain

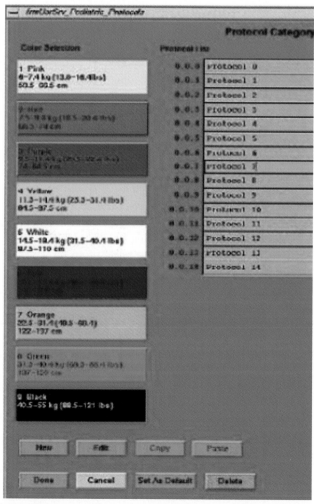

Figure 8.4. Color coding for kids system designed with the goal of reducing radiation dose for pediatric CT scanning. It reduces likelihood of errors in selecting appropriate CT scan protocols based on patient weight and length.

the image noise (*Noise Index*) at a value specified by the user. In this way the dose can be automatically limited in a way that maintains the image quality needed for the clinical diagnostic task. The *AutomA* software uses measured x-ray projection data from a single scout exposure to calculate the patient's attenuation profile within the scanned region to determine the tube current needed to achieve the *Noise Index* selected by the user. The *Noise Index* value approximately equals the standard deviation in the central region of the image when a uniform phantom (similar to the patient's attenuation characteristics) is scanned and reconstructed using the standard reconstruction algorithm. During a scan, *AutomA* dynamically modulates the x-ray tube current value in the longitudinal (z) direction based on the prior calculations from the scout. The *AutomA* software interface also allows the user to specify the maximum and minimum mA range that the system is allowed to use during a scan.

The *Noise Index* is a way to specify the desired image quality. Increasing the value of the *Noise Index* increases the noise in the image and decreases dose. Decreasing the value of the noise index decreases the noise in the image and increases dose. Image noise is one of the most visually conspicuous features in a CT image and therefore selection of *Noise Index* can be correlated to the imaging outcome. Sometimes there is a need to deviate from a pure *Noise Index* value, for example in very large patients where higher noise levels may be acceptable or in very thin patients where a slightly lower noise level may be desired to better visualize the smaller features that may be less conspicuous in thinner patients.

Here are a few additional practical points to consider when using *AutomA*:

(i) The system uses the slice thickness of the first prospective reconstruction prescribed in the study to determine the mA needed to achieve the *Noise Index*. Therefore, if both thick and thin slices are needed for 2D primary reading and for 3D reformation, thick slices with their required *Noise Index* should be the first reconstructed series.

(ii) The system displays a mA table for the prescribed protocol prior to scanning showing the variations of mA in the planned scan. This table should be used to check that the mA values in the scan are in a reasonable range and are not consistently limited by the maximum or minimum mA range setting. This limiting would indicate that the *Noise Index* target might not be achieved and that the dose or noise in this scan may be too high for the imaging needs.

(iii) Although *AutomA* in most cases will reduce the dose compared to a conventional fixed mA scan, in some cases, such as very obese patients, its use could increase the dose if an appropriate maximum mA range has not been set for the protocol.

SmartmA. *SmartmA* (angular or in plane XY modulation) has a different objective than *AutomA*. In anatomy that is highly asymmetric, such as the shoulders, x-rays are significantly less attenuated in anterio-posterior (AP) direction and therefore carry very little noise into the image compared to x-rays in the lateral direction. Thus, the overwhelming abundance of AP x-rays can be substantially reduced without a significant effect on overall image noise. Working in conjunction with *AutomA*, the *SmartmA* feature is a comprehensive three-dimensional mA modulation control that ensures achieving appropriate image quality, as specified by the CT user, at the minimum required radiation dose (Fig. 8.5). As with *AutomA*, the XY modulation for *SmartmA* is determined from a single scout since the patient asymmetry can be computed from the area and amplitude of the projection attenuation.

GE Healthcare's method of using a scout scan to prospectively determine the X, Y and Z mA modulation has some benefits compared to real time methods where the mA modulation is determined from a previous gantry angular position. With a large detector coverage and typical pitch values, the anatomy may change considerably even during half a gantry rotation and the mA value based on prior anatomy may not be optimal for the new anatomy. In

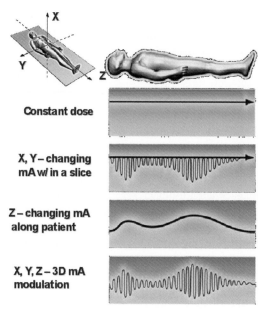

Figure 8.5. Demonstrate the principle of Auto mA and Smart mA method used in GE Healthcare MDCT scanners.

addition, heating or cooling the tube filament modulates the tube current. This thermal inertia of the filament restricts the speed at which the mA can be changed. When mA changes are known in advance, mA commands can be given early to account for the thermal inertia and thereby better synchronize the modulation with the changing anatomy. When mA modulation is predetermined, tube heat load and radiation dose for the upcoming scan can be accurately calculated and displayed before the scan while these important characteristics can only be estimated with a real time method.

Alternative mA Modulation for Sensitive Organs. The ability to modulation the mA has considerable flexibility on GE Healthcare scanners. GE Healthcare is currently developing practical modulation strategies to lower the mA when the x-ray tube is over dose sensitive anterior organs, such as the female breast. Although such modulation may not appear significant on standard dose reports, the patient will receive a useful benefit.

Low kVp, mA Selection and Fast X-ray Switching Time. The use of low kilovolt settings in CT scanning can be an effective way to increase the contrast to noise ratio (CNR) while reducing radiation dose, especially in iodinated contrast enhanced scans in clinical applications to visualize lesions, vascular malformations, tissue blood perfusion and plaque in CT angiography procedures. The reason for this improved efficiency is that the absorption of x-rays by iodine atoms is disproportionately higher for low energy x-ray photons compared to the atoms found in soft body tissues. However, low kVp scanning must be carefully managed with regard to patient size and will usually require increased mA to achieve acceptable results at lower dose than with higher kVp settings. GE Healthcare scanners offer a wide selection of kVp and mA settings to cover a broad range of clinical uses.

The speed at which x-rays are turned on and off may also play a dose reduction role, especially in very short scans such as axial prospectively gated cardiac imaging (GE Healthcare's SnapShot-Pulse) and during ECG based mA modulation. Fast switching enables the acquisition to begin and end together with the radiation, eliminating excessive rise and fall times while data is not acquired.

Dose Reduction in Cardiac Imaging. Retrospectively gated helical coronary CT angiography (CTA) scans can impose a relatively high radiation dose burden. The main reason for the high dose in CTA is that conventional helical scan protocols use very low pitch factors. This is done in order to ensure continuous data availability for the reconstruction of images at each location along the heart at any required heart phase. The low pitch values, typically between 0.3 and 0.18 in 64 row MDCT scanners, result in the x-ray beam irradiating each location along the scan path between 3 to 5 times. However, in many clinical exams, a large portion of the information accumulated during the scan may be discarded since a single-phase reconstruction can often provide the needed diagnostic images for routine cardiac evaluation.

ECG Dose Modulation. When clinically necessary to assure imaging over a broad range of cardiac phases, the most successful method to reduce dose in CTA helical exams is ECG gated x-ray beam current modulation. This method applies high tube current (mA) over a limited range of heart phases to ensure low noise during those phases, while reducing the mA to about 20% or more of the maximum value during the remaining heart phases. Dose reductions of up to 30% to 50% can be achieved compared to a scan without current modulation.

SnapShot-Pulse, Prospectively Gated Cardiac Acquisition. A substantial dose reduction over ECG driven mA modulation is to employ prospectively gated axial scans in which x-rays are turned on only during the required heart phase and turned off completely at all other times. This method can often be used with some caveats when it is clinically not necessary to evaluate heart function. This method is sometimes referred to as a *step-and-shoot* acquisition because the system exposes the patient only when the table is stationary and then the table translates, or "steps," to the next location prior to the next exposure (Fig. 8.6). SnapShot Pulse requires precision x-ray on/off switching, synchronized to exact table movements and to the ECG signal in order to ensure maximum dose reduction and accurate continuity of the acquired data between steps. In addition, image reconstruction algorithms are required to produce high quality thin slice axial images from ECG gated cone beam acquisitions and to provide seamless data transition at the boundaries between scans. Prospectively gated cardiac acquisition is available on the GE Healthcare 64-row or greater MDCT scanners as the *SnapShot-Pulse* scanning mode. The technique takes advantage of the 40-mm-wide detector array with 64 rows of 0.625-mm elements and the advanced axial cone beam reconstruction algorithms to enable complete coverage of any heart in 3 or 4 incremental acquisitions. Studies show that the technique is suitable for the many patients, can reduce dose up to 83% compared to retrospectively gated cardiac scans without ECG mA modulation and that image quality is as good or better than in prospective gating (Fig. 8.7).

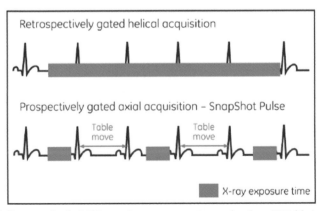

Figure 8.6. Step-and-Shoot method of CT scanning exposes patient only when CT table is stationary and only during part of the heart cycle providing lower dose.

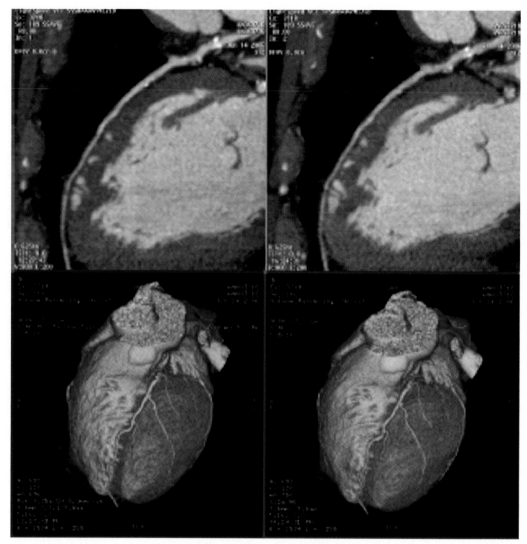

Figure 8.7. Images reconstructed from data acquired with SnapShot-Pulse scanning protocols.

Summary

GE Healthcare provides a wide variety of dose management features to minimize radiation dose during CT scans. CT users are encouraged to become familiar with this array of dose reduction features and employ them whenever clinically appropriate. GE Healthcare offers a variety of training opportunities to use the features to manage patient dose.

Acknowledgements

The authors graciously acknowledge and thank Uri Shreter for outlining and providing the initial information for this chapter. We also acknowledge the inventive genius and dedicated hard work of the GE Healthcare Engineering and Applications teams in bringing to clinical practice the dose reduction and management tools described in this chapter.

Strategies to Reduce Radiation Dose in Philips Multidetector Computed Tomography Scanners
■ **Nirmal K. Soni, PhD and N. Abraham Cohn, Ph.D**

Balancing dose with image quality is a key factor in the development of future CT technologies. Philips Medical Systems has a three-stage approach to patient dose reduction: (i) CT systems are designed with a focus on improving dose efficiency throughout the system; (ii) Multiple current modulation techniques have been developed that retain image quality while reducing dose, and (iii) CT systems are designed to provide more awareness and measurements of radiation usage and dose.

Improved Dose Efficiency

Through technological innovation in the last decade, Philips CT systems have become more dose efficient. These innovations include advancements in beam filtration, detectors, reconstruction, and postprocessing algorithms.

Beam Filtration. Philips Brilliance CT scanners have an internal filtration of 2.5 mm aluminum equivalence at 80 kVp with an added filtration of 1.2 mm of titanium. This filtration makes the beam harder than the previous CT scanner, resulting in a lower skin dose.

Data Acquisition System Technology. Dose efficiency also has been improved through breakthroughs in detector technology. Conventional data acquisition systems collect and distribute image data in analog format, which is highly susceptible to external noise introduced by electronic components, microphonics, cabling, and stray electromagnetic fields. Recently, the gadolinium oxy-sulfide (GOS) crystal array and back illuminated photodiode have been integrated into a single "Tach" chip. This design dramatically reduces the electronic noise of the system by the direct conversion of the photo detector signals to digital format on the chip. The

Tach chip is fabricated with a unique mixed-signal process that entirely isolates the analog and digital sections inside the chip for optimum noise capability. The high sensitivity, high speed, and low-noise capability of Tach provides greater than 1,000,000 to 1 dynamic range. The benefits of using Tach can be summarized as (Fig. 8.8) as follows:

- ■ Lowers dose for large patients
- ■ Enables low-dose screening protocols with excellent image quality
- ■ Improves low contrast resolution
- ■ Maximizes spatial resolution
- ■ Inherently linear response
- ■ Each channel has its own 20-bit A/D converter, eliminating need for multiplexing and therefore reducing possibility of crosstalk. This results in artifact-free imaging (no rings, bands, or streaks)
- ■ Supports more than 2000 views per rotation acquisition independent of rotational speeds, resulting in uncompromised cardiac image quality without streaks and consistent spatial resolution up to edge of the reconstructed field of view.

Image Reconstruction for Helical Cone-Beam CT. The introduction of large z-axis detector coverage (40 mm) requires new techniques for image reconstruction. As increase in cone angle (the angle between the beam edge and the gantry rotation plane) can lead to inconsistencies resulting from the variation of the patient attenuation map along the axis of rotation. These inconsistencies result in cone beam artifacts. One way to minimize cone beam artifacts is by adopting *approximation method* for reconstructing cone beam projections acquired during a helical path of the source-detector system. The *approximate reconstruction methods* are used to handle incomplete source

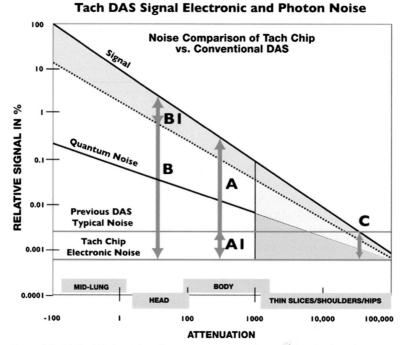

Figure 8.8. Philips' Tech DAS performance. **A:** Scan at the same dose levels and improve Image Quality (S/N ratio) compared to non-Tach systems, **A1:** Represents additional signal gained due to Tach, **B:** Lower the dose and maintain same image quality compared to non-Tach systems, **B1:** Represents the lower dose due to Tach, **C:** Signals that would otherwise be drowned out by noise are detectable with Tach. As a result, Tach extends the range of low-dose applications/anatomy examined with diagnostic Image quality.

trajectories. These are based on a two-dimensional Fourier decomposition of the patient x-ray attenuation map, which makes them simple and computationally more efficient.

Using an approximate method, one can suppress cone beam artifacts by back-projecting only the interpolated readings that lie approximately on an oblique plane that contains the voxel. Unfortunately, from a practical point of view, it is necessary to back-project to each voxel interpolated readings that belong to all the projections that illuminate it. Use of all projections helps improve the dose utility, i.e., reducing the image noise level. The dominant noise mechanism in CT is the Poisson probability function of the photons of each single ray to be absorbed by the patient. In addition full back projection helps reduce the level of image artifacts originating from the patient motion and windmill artifacts originating from an under-sampling along the axis of rotation.

Suppression of cone beam artifacts and achievement of low image noise can be performed simultaneously within the frames of approximate reconstruction methods. The image noise power spectrum (NPS) in CT is concentrated in axial plane at Fourier frequencies that are typically larger than four line pairs per centimeter. However, the cone beam (CB) artifacts contain lower in-plane frequencies. Therefore, to suppress CB artifacts, it is sufficient to obtain the contributions of the low-frequency Fourier components to the image (low frequency image) by using a small angular range of projections that illuminate each voxel. To reduce image noise, one must obtain a high-frequency image by using all the projections illuminating the voxel. The final image is obtained by adding these low- and high-frequency images together.

Eclipse Collimator. The idea behind the eclipse collimator is to reduce the length of irradiated area during a scan by illuminating only those detector rows that contribute to the desired image positions. During a spiral acquisition the areas at the beginning and at the end of the scan contribute significantly to dose. These "overscan" areas can be reduced by closing collimator blades to the extent needed for image reconstruction and opening them in sync as the scan progresses. The blades are closed once again at the end of the scan. Such collimator design is necessary for collimations wider than 40 mm due to the larger opening.

CT Current Selection Techniques

CT current selection and modulation techniques have been developed for the purpose of reducing patient radiation dose and keeping high quality diagnostic value.

Automatic Current Selection. Automatic current selection (ACS) suggests an optimized x-ray tube current for the entire planned scan. This technique uses the scout scan to estimate patient size and water-equivalent attenuation. On the basis of the water equivalent attenuation and an internal protocol reference, the technique provides a suggested 'mAs' for the desired diagnostic purpose. Thus, each patient scan is optimized to achieve the desired image quality (i.e., noise level) with the lowest dose. For example, if the patient attenuation is less than the reference, the algorithm suggests a decrease in the *reference mAs.*

In ACS, each protocol has a baseline mAs associated with a reference database. Because different image quality is required for various protocols, each protocol has its own stored reference. After a scout scan image is acquired, the projection data is processed to smooth out sharp variations for the equivalent size calculation. The projection data at a couch position is one dimensional and is not enough for the accurate calculation of the cross section of the patient. However, the maximum thickness of the patient can be estimated quite accurately. An ellipse or circular model generally is used to describe the cross section of the patient and to estimate the length of the long/short axes.

To select the right mAs for desired diagnostics after computing patient equivalent size, standard noise levels of clinical protocols must be first established that are equivalent to standard patient sizes. The calculated patient size is then compared with the standard size to determine scan mAs that can deliver same level of image quality as defined in the protocol. If the calculated size is larger or smaller than the standard size of the protocol, the suggested mAs will be higher or lower than the protocol mAs, respectively. ACS usually provides features that allow users to select different noise levels according to the requirements of the diagnostics and dose savings. The mAs selection of the ACS depends on the protocol setting, model calculation, noise level selection, and diagnostic requirements. Usually the noise level selection provides quite a wide range that covers different requirements of image quality and dose saving. Default standard noise levels of clinical protocols provide general references for the automatic selection of scan mAs. When the user overrides the mAs, the reference database is automatically updated and adjusted to learn from the user's preferences.

As part of the ACS tool performance investigations, 40 patients were scanned in two different sites (in Carmel Medical Center, Israel, and Angers University Hospital, France) on the Mx8000IDT (64-row MDCT) with the use of a nominal abdomen protocol. The saved reference image had a value of 34.5 cm of water equivalent weighted diameter. It can be clearly observed from Figure 8.9 that the noise variation versus the weighted diameter is much larger when the ACS function is turned off.

Dynamic Dose Modulation. The optimized x-ray tube current at a path i is proportional to the square root of the attenuation along the path:

$$(mA)_i \propto \sqrt{A_i}$$

where A_i is the attenuation along the X-ray path i. The difference in the attenuations of the X-rays through different paths can be quite large. For example, when the tube rotates around the shoulders, the direction across the shoulders has much larger attenuation then the direction perpendicular it. Thus, when the x-ray tube rotates

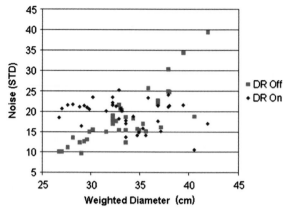

Figure 8.9. Results of an ACS related research of 40 patients in two different hospitals. The noise is plotted as a function of the patient weighted diameter for scans using the ACS tool (DR on) and without using the ACS tool (DR off).

around a subject, the current modulation can be quite large and beyond the capability of the most generators. To solve this problem a less-optimized format of dose modulation generally is used where the mA is no longer proportional to the square root of the attenuation, but to A^α where α is a positive number smaller than 0.5.

Angular dynamic dose modulation (DDOM) modulates x-ray tube current during the scan according to the size of scanned object. During a helical scan, projection data is acquired at each source angular position. These data are filtered and processed to determine the maximum attenuation of the patient at the given source angular position. DDOM uses previously measured attenuation to predict tube current at a source position 180 or 360 degrees from the latest source angular position. Because of the latency of the tube/generator system, caution must be exercised to ensure that the required mA is delivered to the correct source angular position. The dose savings of the DDOM depend on the shape of the object under scan. If a cylindrical water phantom is scanned at the isocenter of the scanner, there is no current modulation or dose saving. Clinical studies show that the dose saving is approximately 10% for head scan and 20–40% for chest scan depending on the patient.

Longitudinal Dose Modulation. The modulation of the mAs along the longitudinal axis (z-axis) of the patient or along the bed is called Z-DOM (Fig. 8.10). This dose modulation controls the uniformity of the image quality along the patient's longitudinal axis. Z-DOM is a low-frequency modulation that modulates the tube current according to the changes in the body attenuation along z.

The motivation of using Z-DOM is twofold: (i) reduce dose to the patient in organs in which the attenuation is lower because lower dose is sufficient to provide desired diagnostic image quality and (ii) maintain uniform image quality within the scan.

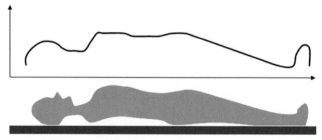

Figure 8.10. The Z-Dose Modulation, a schematic view.

Without using Z-Dom, the mAs is constant and the noise varies significantly as a function of the organ attenuation (water equivalent diameter) along the scan (Fig. 8.11, dashed line). Using Z-Dom, the noise is planned to vary only slightly (or not at all) as a function of the organ water equivalent diameter along the scan (Fig. 8.11, solid line). The variation of the noise along the scan can be determined by a dedicated noise factor. In Figure 8.11, it can be observed that there is a slight variation in the noise with the change of the organ diameter (attenuation). If the noise factor is set to 1 the noise is uniform.

Before the Z-DOM scan, a scout scan is performed. The data are then processed and a weighted water equivalent diameter is estimated along the longitudinal axis (z). The protocol mAs can be set by the user or by the ACS function. The protocol mAs shown to the user is the maximal mAs in the scan to be performed according to the regulations. The average and the minimal mAs of the planned scan are displayed as well. The mAs profile along z is calculated using the maximum mAs and the pre-calculated weighted diameter. It also takes into account the tube characteristics along with the specific scan parameters.

The use of Z-DOM along with ACS improves the noise uniformity between patients and longitudinally for a single patient while keeping the dose lower especially in smaller patients and for less attenuating organs (i.e., the lungs). For abdomen protocols the average mAs of the modulated profiles is lower by ~32% than the maximum profile mAs (within a patient).

Dose Savings in Cardiac CT. Because the purpose of a cardiac scan is to track dynamic pulsing coronaries, a high temporal resolution scan is vital. The common way to achieve a sufficient temporal resolution in a cardiac scan is to apply a multicycle reconstruction mode. In this mode each image is reconstructed from several successive cardiac cycles and each cycle contributes limited data around a (relatively) quiet phase of the heart. Two system properties are used to provide qualitative data for such a reconstruction mode: (i) a high tube current, which reduces noise in the typical strict 180-degree reconstruction mode, and (ii) a low pitch scan, which is used to capture a large number of phase points for the multicycle reconstruction. Both of these properties result in a high amount of dose.

Several methods have been developed to cope with the high dose problem but perhaps the most effective ones rely on a prospective x-ray triggering principle. This principle is intuitive and simple: because the heart motion is periodic, the quiet phases of the heart can be predicted from its monitored history and the system can be directed to turn the x-rays *ON* during the quite phases and *OFF* anywhere else. Implementation of such an idea into a product was introduced in Philips Brilliance 2.0 version under the title Cardiac Dose Modulation. In this scan mode, the tube current is modulated such that for the quiet phase(s) the current is raised to its maximum value (100%) and 20% elsewhere. This scan type provided a dose reduction

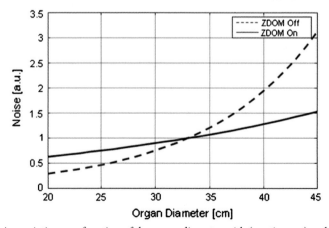

Figure 8.11. The noise variation as a function of the organ diameter with (continuous) and without (dash) using Z-DOM.

of up to ~50% compared with a typical cardiac scan.

The helical dose-modulation strategy with cardiac phase suits a large population of cardiac CT patients but it seems to fail whenever heart rate irregularities appear. Therefore, Philips has a new cardiac axial scan mode that applies prospective triggering mechanism to synchronize irradiation times with the heart's quiet phase. When an arrhythmia is traced, an online algorithm is applied to keep the patient couch in the same position to compensate for this bad scan. This advanced axial scan mode introduces a low-dose scan profile (~75% dose saving compared to a typical helix scan) with an on-line adaptive capability. The benefits of this axial prospective scan mode are only expected to grow in the scope of next generations' scanners which are expected to provide scan coverage large enough to capture the entire heart in a single axial scan.

Summary

Philips Medical Systems provides many tools in its CT scanners that enable optimization of dose reduction while at the same time providing good quality images. Philips displays CT dose descriptors such as CTDI$_{vol}$ and dose length product on the operators console for all scan-protocols and all scan conditions, allowing the customers to assess their dose usage. In addition, to help the customer fully understand the features of the scanner, Philips provides customer education through operator documentation, on-site applications training, off-site classroom training, manufacturer specific publications, customer meetings, and computer-based training.

With the recent increase in CT scanning procedures, there is concern about the impact of the increased radiation dose to the exposed population. Philips is committed to keeping patient doses ALARA ("as low as reasonably achievable") and continues to explore methods of providing excellent image quality while reducing patient dose. In keeping with the ALARA principle, scan technique factors should be chosen to use the minimum patient dose for the desired diagnostic quality of the exam.

Acknowledgments

The information presented in this section has been compiled with significant contribution from the following physicists at Philips Medical Systems: Nirmal K. Soni, PhD, N. Abraham Cohn, PhD, Shmuel Glasberg, PhD, Peter C. Johnson, Eran Langzam, PhD, Zhongmin Lin, PhD, Hugh T. Morgan, PhD, Galit Naveh, PhD, Mark Pepelea, PhD, Iris Sabo-Nabadensky, PhD, Gilad Shechter, PhD, Efrat Shefer, PhD, and Chris Vrettos.

Strategies to Reduce Radiation Dose in Siemens MDCT Scanners
■ Christoph Suess, PhD

Siemens has been in the forefront of technological innovations in CT and has constantly strived to design dose-efficient CT scanners by developing several strategies to reduce radiation dose.

Scanner Design

Many components of CT systems influence the dose efficiency. First, the flat filters located in the tube-collimator assembly add a very important contribution to dose reduction. Our scanners always have had strong flat filters between 5.5 and 11 mm of aluminum equivalent, which is largely higher than the legal requirement of at least 2.5 mm aluminum. This additional filtration requires slightly higher tube load but reduces the dose significantly without impairing the image noise, especially for larger objects. In addition, our scanners adopted shaped filters to reduce the dose in the periphery of the fan beam by a factor of 10 to 15 and not limit the scan field of view.

Highly efficient x-ray detectors are prerequisites for low-dose imaging. The UFC (Ultra Fast Ceramic) material used in all Siemens CT scanner detectors is optimized to ensure extremely short afterglow times and enabling sampling rates up to 5 kHz without any need for afterglow corrections. The same holds for scatter radiation. Any additional correction of measured data would increase noise. To avoid this detriment, Siemens detectors have scatter collimators made of 100-micron thick tungsten sheets with slot ratios of up to 20 for each detector element. Even with Siemen's 64-slice scanners with large z-coverage and accordingly high scatter ratios, there is no need for a postprocessing scatter correction that would impair image quality and dose efficiency.

A major contribution to undesired patient dose in MDCT scanners can be caused by the axial overbeaming, which reduces the axial dose efficiency (z-efficiency) of a CT scanner and increases the CTDI values and patient dose for multislice settings. All Siemens SOMATOM CT scanners since 1995 have a real-time control of the tube collimator and allows to adjust them precisely within a 20-micron interval even during the scan. The new STRATON x-ray tube eliminates the undesired focal spot z-motion caused by the rotating anode with a real-time control system inside the tube assembly. These technical measures keep the overbeaming effects in multiple- and single-row detector CT scanners at the lowest levels defined by the basic physics principals and not by hardware limitations.

Often during the spiral (helical) scan mode, the data acquisition demands a certain amount of data acquired outside the reconstructable volume, the so-called *overscan*. The development of dynamic collimators for the tube allows the avoidance of this undesired effect. The collimator is partly closed at the beginning of the helical scan, opens during the first rotation and, at the end, again closes during the last rotation. Modern high-speed scanners with rotation times down to 0.3 s require very fast and precise collimator mechanics and control systems, and a perfect coordination with the table movement. With such systems the dose e.g. for a 100 mm

spiral scan can be reduced by 35% and by 25% for cardiac H exams.

Data and Image Processing for Noise Reduction. Special adaptive filtering of raw data and images help to reduce noise and dose levels. Siemens SOMATOM CT scanners have different types of adaptive filters for projection data. These filters combine data of different detector elements within a single row (linear filter) or, in multiple row systems, add filtering within rows to reduce the noise in certain types of projection data (2D-Filter).

Siemens have implemented a new type of noise reduction algorithms that work on all type of data sets. By analyzing the image structures, the effect on spatial resolution is minimized, linear variances are calculated for numerous directions in the three-dimensional image space to explore the local morphological properties and determine orientation of edges. Different filters are used, generating three intermediate data sets: a fixed two-dimensional axial convolution implemented as frequency domain filter with freely selectable kernel, an adaptive one-dimensional convolution in direction of the minimal variance and an adaptive one-dimensional convolution in direction of the cross variance.

Depending on the local distribution of variances, intermediate data are mixed by means of local weights. This allows in obtaining an optimally adapted overall filter with minimized noise and least deterioration of information.

The phantom studies indicated noise reduction of up to 40% without affecting the delineation of small structures or edges. The sharpness-to-noise ratio therefore can be improved to the same degree. In clinical cases, dose could be reduced by up to 30% without loss of diagnostically relevant information. The developed algorithm represents a computationally efficient noise reduction with a high potential for dose reduction in CT. Currently such filters are routinely used in cardiac imaging, low dose screening procedures and dual energy applications.

Dose Information for CT Users. Siemens introduced the display of CT dose index ($CTDI_{vol}$) for all their scanners in 1997, because it best visualizes the impact on patient dose of all design and scan parameters like x-ray filters, beam collimation, axial overbeaming and the amount of 'over scan' in spiral CT volume scans.

Siemens started in 1999 to supply information on CTDI and effective dose for all standard protocols delivered with our scanners. The data were calculated with a Monte Carlo program that accounts for all important scanner data like flat and shaped filters, tube voltage, collimator settings and x-ray geometry.

Optimization of Scan Protocols for Clinical Applications and Patient Size. Siemens offer a large variety of predefined clinical protocols for all kinds of CT applications. First of all, the kVp need to be adjusted to the object size and the expected tissue contrasts, the mAs together with the kV and the detector collimation define the patient dose level and the noise in the measured projection data. Even for a certain dose level, the image characteristics may be balanced to a high degree between the spatial resolution and image noise by the convolution kernel in the filtered back projection. The Siemens SOMATOM range of CT scanners offer a set of more than 100 different clinical scan protocols including a detailed description of the scan parameters and the diagnostic aspects.

Optimization of Pediatric Scan Protocols. Especially in pediatric scanning, the mAs must be modified over a wide range to adapt for the variations in patient size. For routine use, Siemens have found it most convenient and safe to base the adapted pediatric protocols on the patient's weight and age. For head imaging, Siemens chose four different age groups because the attenuation in the head depends mainly on the ossification of the skull, which develops by age and almost reaches adult levels after the age of 6 years.

In the chest and abdomen of pediatric patients, the attenuation of calcified tissues plays a minor role. The main factor is the thickness of the penetrated soft tissues, best represented by the patient's weight. Therefore, Siemens chose six different weight groups to define the mAs steps, starting with 15% of the adult mAs for children weighing less than 15 kg (Table 8.1). With these charts the mAs and therefore radiation dose can be reduced up to a factor of four in the scanning of pediatric heads and up to a factor of seven for abdomen and pelvis scans. These settings should be further reduced for scans that don't require the full image quality, for example in the follow-up studies.

The optimization of tube voltage was an important issue in the early days of CT. Lower kV settings increase the contrast of bone, iodine, and some soft tissues, but the x-ray output significantly reduces with lower tube potential. Especially in pediatric applications, smaller volumes are scanned at moderate or low tube loadings, which would allow for low kVp settings. Image quality in CT should be specified as image noise and contrast, assuming constant spatial resolution.

Comparing only image noise and dose for 80 kVp and 120 kVp in small objects, simulating

	Table 8.1	Recommended mAs settings for adapted pediatric protocols; data are given for Somatom Sensation 64, but the relation of mAs settings is valid for all Siemens scanners

Weight classes, kg	Thorax scans, mAs, % of adult settings	Abdomen/pelvic scans, mAs, % of adult settings
<15	15	15
15–24	25	25
25–34	40	35
35–44	60	50
45–54	80	75
>54	100	100

The settings for children weighing less than 15 kg are routinely reduced to just 25 mAs for abdomen and 15 mAs for thorax scans, i.e., 15% of the adult settings.

children up to 45 kg, there is not much difference between the two, which means that both could be used without dose penalty. When examining the dose, image noise, and iodine contrast, the 80-kVp scans show a 40% increase of the signal-to-noise ratio, which allows the operator to cut the dose by half for contrast-enhanced pediatric studies. Siemens SOMATOM CT pediatric scan protocols use the low kVp for all CT angiograms. Many institutions have extended the 80-kVp setting to all their pediatric contrast studies. The operator even can apply lower kVp to reduce dose levels in adult CT exams like carotid CT angiograms or, in slim patients, cardiac CTA in slim patients.. The optimization of the preprogrammed pediatric protocols with respect to mA settings and tube voltage selection has led to a dose reduction on all Siemens MDCT scanners. Beside the scanner design and application considerations, the most promising latest technical innovations with a wide range of clinical applications are the tube current modulation and the automatic exposure control.

Tube Current Modulation. For several decades it was state-of-the-art in CT to scan at constant kVp and mA settings, although the patient's attenuation may change dramatically during a single spiral scan. In the 1990s, the investigation on the noise propagation in the image reconstruction process illustrated that the pixel noise in the CT image was found to be dominated by the projections with high attenuation and, accordingly, high noise levels of the measured data. To compensate for this effect, to balance the noise for the different projection angles and to minimize dose for a certain image noise level, it was suggested to modulate the tube current proportional to the square root of attenuation. For all noncircular cross sections, the modulated primary radiation intensity promised to achieve the desired image quality at dose levels reduced by 10–50%.

Online Adaptive Angular Current Modulation: "CARE Dose". The preprogrammed sinusoidal mA-modulation with only 50% amplitude demonstrated no significant advantages compared with the conventional constant current approach, whereas the different implementation

on Siemens SOMATOM CT scanners with an attenuation based online current modulation featuring amplitudes of more than 90% showed great potential for dose reduction in phantom studies and in several clinical trials. The potential of dose reduction of 10–50% motivated Siemens to invest on the fast tube current modulation in the 1990s and to implement the attenuation based on-line current modulation CARE Dose on all scanners as a basic feature.

Since then the technical performance of Siemens *SOMATOM CT* generators and tubes has been improved dramatically to cope with the demands of the latest high-end cardiac CT scanners. The modern high-frequency transformers in Siemens scanners can easily provide the essential accuracy of tube potential and the desired high speed of current variation. By keeping the capacities of the generator-cable-tube assembly very low and the current control circuits very fast and efficient, Siemens meanwhile can change the tube load from 80 kW down to 3 kW in just 30 ms and vice-versa in the same time frame.

This change, of course, puts strong demands on the tube cathode. Conventional solenoidal filaments would not sustain this fast heating and the thermal inertia would not allow for fast lowering of tube current. Our new STRATON tube has a flat emitter that provides these essential features for ultra-fast current modulation. With these technical innovations Siemens implemented a series of different clinical applications that use the current modulation to reduce dose to the patient and, for certain types of exams, to the physician.

Angular Tube Current Modulation: "Hand" CARE. Beside the attenuation-based current modulation, a preprogrammed angular current modulation reduces dose in several different types of CT exams. For many CT-guided interventional procedures, even with relatively low exposure rates, the time-consuming interventions may produce high dose levels to the patient and to the physician. To reduce this dose, Siemens introduced the angular modulation *Hand CARE*, which reduces or even switches off the radiation for three different angular segments of the scan: AP and left or right decubitus. This type of modulation reduces the effective dose to the patient by 35% and dose to the physician's hands up to 72%. This technique is widely accepted on Siemens scanners because it still provides the desired real-time imaging with a sufficient frame rate of two images per second without any loss of image quality. A similar approach, the "organ-based" current modulation, can be used to care for certain sensitive organs like the eye lens or the female breast. Early results on thoracic imaging indicated reduction in breast dose by 30–40% without any compromise in image quality. These types of pre-programmed or on-line rotational tube current modulation can be extended and optimized to fully achieve AEC.

Automatic Exposure Control: "CARE Dose 4D". Siemens began in the mid 1990s to investigate automatic approaches to evaluate the patient's size and attenuation during the examination and adjust the scan parameters accordingly. Because each CT exam starts with a scout-scan, the projection data from these scans are used to detect the patient's attenuation for the selected viewing angle, in most cases AP or lateral. With some elaborate algorithms Siemens succeeded to predict the attenuation perpendicular to this projection angle with an error of less than 20%. Knowing the AP and lateral attenuation at every axial position of the scan, one can predict the image quality for a certain exposure or, vice versa, set the right exposure to yield the desired image quality for every slice.

The issue of the best image quality for different patient sizes and organ regions was unresolved. As is known from x-ray imaging systems, the AEC tries to maintain a constant signal at the image receptor which, for CT, would result in a constant noise for all the reconstructed images of a scan. That first idea was tested in phantom experiments but proved to be impractical and actually not desirable for diagnostic image quality. CT image noise can best be tested and demonstrated in uniform water phantoms of different sizes. Noise results for a series of cylindrical water phantoms with diameters ranging from 10 cm to 40 cm, scanned with different mAs, are presented in Table 8.2.

The typical settings of, for example, 150 mAs for a normal abdomen with a 30-cm diameter result in a noise level of 14 HU. Scanning this series of phantoms with these constant mAs, one would receive noise levels between 1.9 HU for the smallest phantom and 38 HU for the 40 cm, which of course is not adequate with respect to dose for the small phantoms and image noise for the large phantoms. Following the "constant noise" approach, as shown in the third row of Table 8.2, one would like to preserve the same noise level of 14 HU in all sections and would have to apply more than 1100 mAs for the 40-cm phantom and just 2.7 mAs for the smallest diameter. Although available on modern CT scanners, such settings with extensive patient exposure for large or unacceptable noise levels for small cross sections are not used in diagnostic CT scans with standard image-quality requirements.

Table 8.2	Exposure levels and image noise for different size water phantoms					
Phantom diameter, cm	10	14	20	25	**30**	40
Image noise (HU) for a scan with 150 mAs	1.9	2.8	5.2	8.5	**14**	38
mAs for constant image noise (14 HU)	*2.7*	*6.1*	20	55	**150**	*1108*
CARE Dose 4D "adapted" mAs setting	**20**	**30**	**55**	**91**	**150**	**290**
CARE Dose 4D resulting image noise	5.2	6.3	8.5	10.9	**14**	27.4

A typical setting of 150 mAs for a normal abdomen with 30-cm diameter results in a noise level of 14 HU. Scanning the series of phantoms with these constant mAs, noise levels vary between 1.9 HU for the smallest phantom and 38 HU for the 40 cm, which of course is not adequate with respect to dose for the small phantoms and image noise for the large phantoms. Following the "constant noise" approach of other manufacturers, third row of the table, one would apply more than 1100 mAs for the 40 cm phantom and just 2.7 mAs for the smallest diameter. The moderate adaptation of mAs by the Siemens exposure control CARE Dose 4D delivers adequate mAs (shown bold on 4th row) to produce diagnostic noise levels in all sizes of phantoms and patients.

A series of simulation and clinical studies was necessary to define the exposure and image quality levels adequate for diagnostic needs. At several clinical sites Siemens used standard exams and added noise to the scan data to simulate lower exposure and greater noise levels. With these trials the acceptable noise levels for many different types of organs and a large variation of patient sizes and, of course, different radiologists were evaluated. Although the radiologists had varying expectations for image quality, i.e., the noise levels, the relative noise favored for the different phantom and patient size was rather constant. This experience led Siemens to the concept of selecting typical, in other words reference mAs, which are used for normal patients, and adjust the mAs for different patient attenuation according to a rather moderate exponential function with exponent 0.5 for smaller and 0.33 for larger objects (Fig. 8.12).

This rather pragmatic approach was not easy to argue from a theoretical point of view, but it appeared very practical because it reflected the state of the art in clinical CT scanning and generated the image quality people expected. For pediatric scans, the automatically adjusted mAs settings were very close to the manually optimized protocols (Table 8.1) and, for obese patients, resulting mAs matched nicely with the clinical charts evaluated by experienced users. Meanwhile, many clinical studies validated the concept of this type of AEC (CARE Dose 4D).

The resulting dose reduction is favored by the combination of absolute mAs adaptation to patient size, fast and highly dynamic axial and rotational mA modulation, which is based on the real-time information on patient attenuation acquired in the CT detector system (Fig. 8.13). CARE Dose 4D was introduced in 2003 and currently about 90% of all Siemens clinical scans are performed with AEC to achieve improved desired diagnostic image quality at lowest dose levels.

Dose Reduction in Cardiac CT

With the introduction of MDCT scanners rotating at less than 500 ms, imaging of the heart at

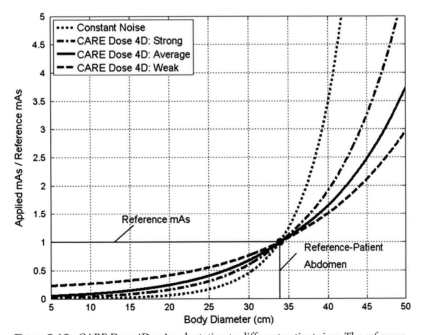

Figure 8.12. CARE Dose 4D mAs adaptation to different patient sizes. The *reference mAs* for a typical normal patient (33 cm diameter) are defined by the user. The AEC adapts the mAs to the different object sizes rather moderate (solid line) compared with the constant noise approach (dotted line). Different slopes for the modulation curve can be selected (dashed lines) in the system.

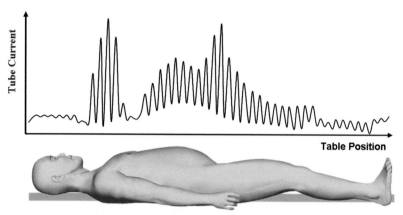

Figure 8.13. CARE Dose 4D on-line mA modulation during a whole body spiral scan. The high dynamic range for angular and z-axis tube current modulation delivers optimal exposure levels to the different organs in one scan. Especially in the shoulders and pelvis the angular modulation reduces the patient dose and improves the image quality.

reasonable spatial and temporal resolution became feasible. However, shortly after the introduction of cardiac spiral scanning, the greater dose levels raised discussions about the risk versus benefit of cardiac CT. Siemens applied an ECG-related tube current modulation to significantly reduce patient exposure. For all data segments not used to reconstruct the high quality angiographic images in the diastolic phase, the tube current was reduced to 25% of its nominal value. This so-called *ECG-Pulsing* of the tube current was reported to reduce patient dose in cardiac CT by up to 50%, depending on the patient's heart rate. Controlled studies on larger cohorts of cardiac patients demonstrated an average dose reduction of 45% and 48% in women and men, respectively.

With technical advances extending the number of slices to 16 and then 64, and the faster rotation of scanners down to 0.4 and 0.33 s, the spatial and temporal resolution was increasing dramatically, but thinner slices and shorter reconstruction intervals required an increase in tube output, causing greater exposure and patient dose levels. A study for a cohort of 1035 patients reported an effective dose of 6.4 mSv for the 16-slice scanner and 11.0 mSv for the 64-slice scanner run in constant tube current mode.

With the use of ECG-controlled mA-modulation and 100 kVp in slim patients, the dose could be reduced between 37% and 64%, coming down to moderate exposure levels significantly below 5 mSv.

Despite these technical advances, the limited temporal resolution between 165 and 200 ms causes problems imaging at higher heart rates, which required the administration of beta-blockers for cardiac CT scanning. The use of multiple segment reconstruction may help to improve spatial resolution, but it requires a very stable heart rate to avoid inconsistent data and very low pitch values, again causing high dose levels. The desirable temporal resolution of less than 100 ms in single-segment reconstruction, essential to scan at greater heart rates, would require gantry rotation times below 200 ms far beyond the capabilities of state-of-the-art mechanical scanner concepts.

This limitation brought up the idea of multiple x-ray sources scanning simultaneously and cutting the temporal resolution by half. The technical concept proved to be practical, but scanning with 2 × 80 kW might of course deliver two times the exposure of a single source system. On the world's first commercial Dual-Source MDCT scanner, the Siemens SOMA-TOM Definition implemented various measures to limit the dose and, finally, ended up with even lower exposure levels than the conventional single-source MDCT scanners.

First of all, the x-ray beam was optimized for cardiac applications. All scanners use shaped filters to reduce dose and adapt the x-ray flux to the non-uniform patient attenuation. However, in cardiac CT the situation is very different. Only the rather small organ in the center of the thorax defines the region of interest for this examination; details outside are not of primary interest. A very aggressive shaped filter was implemented to almost block radiation outside the cardiac field of view. The effect on dose reduction can best be expressed by the different weighted CTDI values. Although for standard body exams the scanner delivers a $CTDI_{vol}$ of 7.2 mGy per 100 mAs, the dose index and, accordingly, the patient dose for cardiac scans reduces by 21% down to just 5.7 mGy per 100 mAs.

The dose levels in cardiac scans mainly suffer from the very low pitch values. For heart rates up to typically 60 bpm, pitch values of 0.18 to 0.22 are needed to image the heart at a certain phase without gaps. At higher heart rates, the pitch could be increased proportional to the heart rate still maintaining the full coverage. Single-source scanners cannot take advantage of that relationship because of their limited temporal resolution. The dual-source CT system, however, has a very high and constant temporal resolution of 83 ms, i.e., one-fourth the rotation time, which allows

one to increase the cardiac pitch up to 0.5 for heart rates beyond 100 bpm and reduce the dose by 60% compared with a pitch of 0.2 that is normally used on single-source MDCT scanners even for higher heart rates.

ECG pulsing is also implemented on this type of CT scanner. It is, in our opinion, essential and in general more efficient on dual-source MDCT scanners because only 90 degrees of projection data are needed and the dose can be kept at low levels for a long period of the cardiac cycle. With the SOMATOM Definition, it is further optimized with the introduction of fast ramping of the tube current: 20–30 ms ramp from 500 to 100 mA and vice-versa. An automated real-time detection of extra-systoles during the scan allows one to switch tube current on even in patients with suspected irregular heart rates. In these cases the current is kept at high level during the extra-systole and low noise images can be reconstructed at any interval of this cardiac cycle. This new kind of implementation allows the use of pulsing to reduce patient dose in all kind of cardiac exams.

These combined measures significantly reduce the dose levels. Depending on the patient's heart rate and the type of scan mode chosen, the dose comes down to 50% or less compared to a standard single source CT scanner for cardiac exams. Figure 8.14 demonstrates the dose reduction for the different heart rates, associated with the various technical innovations implemented on the SOMATOM Definition.

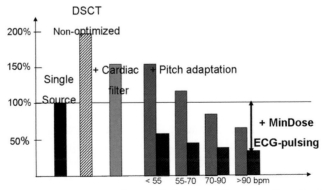

Figure 8.14. Cardiac dose for SOMATOM Definition dual-source CT scanner. Several technical features were implemented to reduce the cardiac dose from the theoretical value of twice the dose of a single source down to even less than 50% of the single source dose. Especially for higher heart rates, the higher pitch values and the very efficient tube current modulation MinDose brings dose down to the levels of the step-and-shoot cardiac scans.

Whenever a functional study of the heart is not required, the data outside the CTA reconstruction interval are not essential for diagnosis. In these cases, we further reduce the tube current down to 4% of the nominal value (ECG pulsing MinDose) or completely switch off the tube current, which results in the cardiac step-and-shoot scan mode. Both techniques result in similar dose levels, which can be as low as 2 mSv for certain cases scanned at 100 kV tube potential. Although this step-and-shoot mode with very low exposure levels is restricted to low heart rates in single-source scanners, it can be used for all heart rates in dual-source machines. These new concepts further push for the low dose cardiac CT examinations.

Future Innovations

The technical advances of the recent years brought a remarkable dose reduction for all types of CT examinations, but further steps can be expected. Siemens works on new detector concepts, which can separate the energy information in the x-ray spectra. These new types of detectors open up new imaging mechanisms, allow to enhance tissue contrasts and to deliver diagnostic image quality at even lower dose levels. With the dramatic advances of computational power, further essential steps can also be expected from advanced algorithms for noise reduction working on projection data in three dimensions and, for dynamic studies, even in four-dimensional space. Various algorithms for volume or cone beam CT image reconstruction emerged in the recent years. New reconstruction algorithms, like for instance the iterative reconstruction, definitely have the potential to reduce radiation dose, increase spatial resolution, and reduce image noise almost independently. Although in clinical use now for several decades, CT still is open for essential future innovations to further improve image quality and reduce patient dose levels.

Acknowledgments

I want to thank my colleagues Dr. Andreas Schaller for the fruitful technical discussions and David Mathieson for reviewing the article.

Strategies to Reduce Radiation Dose in Toshiba Multiple-row Detector Computed Tomography Scanners
■ Richard Mather, PhD

To adhere to the ALARA principle and always put patient safety first, Toshiba Medical Systems has designed its CT scanners to give the best image quality at the lowest possible dose. From the dual-supported anode x-ray tube to the ultra-efficient quantum detector system and noise-free DAS, to the dose-saving ^{SURE}Exposure3D tube current (mA) modulation software, to advanced, adaptive reconstruction and noise reduction algorithms, the Aquilion system is designed to deliver the best image quality at the lowest possible dose.

Quantum Detectors

An acquisition system containing detectors and electronics that perform well under low-signal conditions forms the foundation of a dose-efficient scanner. At the core of the Quantum Detector is Toshiba's patented illumination detector material. Through a proprietary manufacturing process, praseodymium-doped gadolinium oxy-sulfide (GOS) crystals are sintered into a highly efficient CT detector. The illumination material has an absorption efficiency of greater than 99% and is optically transparent with light output 2.3 times that of cadmium tungstate ($CdWO_4$). It is characterized by fast decay times and low afterglow properties that allow artifact-free scanning down to less than 0.35 s per rotation and below. Combined with precise and highly shielded electronics to ensure the quietest, truest signal possible, the Quantum

Detectors ensure maximum signal in low dose acquisitions.

MegaCool Tube

Vibrations in the anode of the x-ray tube can cause instabilities in the x-ray beam that necessitate wider collimation and thus increase penumbra and radiation dose. Toshiba designed its MegaCool x-ray tube with bearing supports on both ends of the anode axis. This improves anode and beam stability, allowing high-quality imaging to be performed at fast rotation speeds, up to 0.35 s per rotation, while minimizing extra patient dose from penumbra. Furthermore, the MegaCool tube has an innovative feature to collect off-focal electrons and prevent them from producing x-rays. If these off-focal electrons are not captured, the x-rays created by them can lead to artifacts, image quality degradation, as well as unnecessary patient dose. By fitting a positively charged grid near the electrically grounded anode, any secondary, off-focal electrons are captured and removed from the system. In this way, the MegaCool tube provides optimum image quality with a minimum of radiation dose to the patient.

^{SURE}Exposure3D

Since the human body is neither perfectly round nor uniform in size and density, different mAs settings are required to achieve uniform image quality throughout different parts of the body. Toshiba's ^{SURE}Exposure3D software automatically adapts the mAs based on actual patient size and rapidly adjusts the mAs during the scan to adapt to and compensate for all of these changes in attenuation level. Using data from the AP and lateral scout scans, the software determines exactly how much mAs is necessary to maintain a user-defined level of image quality (Fig. 8.15). ^{SURE}Exposure3D adjusts the mAs with respect to all three dimensions (x, y, and z). Therefore, as the scan moves from the shoulders to the lung, the mAs goes down, and as the tube rotates around the patient, less mAs is used anterior-posterior than laterally. For the same image quality level, compared to non-modulated scanning, ^{SURE}Exposure3D can reduce the dose by up to 40%.

The unique nature of coronary imaging gives another opportunity for dose savings via tube current (mA) modulation techniques. With low and steady heart rates, the optimum phase for

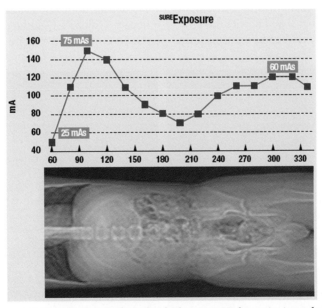

Figure 8.15. ^{SURE}Exposure tailors the dose to the individual patient. Higher mAs, is needed to penetrate dense areas like the upper abdomen and bony pelvis while lower mAs is adequate in less-dense areas like the lung. Overall dose can be lowered by as much as 40% while preserving uniform image quality.

reconstruction is typically between 65% and 80% of the R-R cycle. Because the data in the rest of the cardiac cycle is used only for examining the bulk ventricular function, a much lower mAs value is necessary when acquiring this portion of the data. ^{SURE}Exposure3D with ECG dose modulation allows the tube current (mA) to be significantly reduced during the systolic phases of the cardiac cycle, enabling a reduction in patient dose of as much as 50%.

Boost^{3D}

Even with an optimized detector system and mAs modulation, highly attenuating anatomy such as the shoulders and pelvis can create deficits in the number of photons reaching the detectors. This localized reduction in photon count degrades image quality in the form of excess noise and streak artifacts. Historically, these artifacts could only be combated by increasing the mAs and tube voltage (kVp) to overcome the low photon counts. However, because increasing the imaging technique results in greater patient dose, Toshiba engineers developed an adaptive, three-dimensional algorithm that preferentially corrects the raw data in areas with low photon count. This algorithm, called *Boost^{3D}*, seeks out portions of the raw-projection data where there is a disproportionate loss in x-ray signal and applies the three-dimensional filter locally, thereby reducing image noise and streak artifacts. In areas of normal signal, no correction is applied, and the native image quality is preserved.

Such local, or adaptive, techniques produce the optimum results because the filter is applied only where it is needed. Furthermore, because this algorithm mitigates the effects of photon starvation, it can be applied either to enhance images using conventional mAs settings, or to allow low-dose imaging with acceptable image quality by reducing the scan technique and, thereby, reducing the patient dose. Figure 8.16A demonstrates images through the shoulder in a cardiac bypass patient using a relatively low scan technique. The images exhibit typical structured noise and streak artifacts resulting from the low photon count. However, when Boost^{3D} is applied, the image noise is greatly reduced and the streak artifacts disappear (Figure 8.16B). By reducing the noise and mitigating the effects of low-dose scanning, adaptive techniques such as Boost^{3D} are key developments in Toshiba's commitment to patient focused imaging.

Quantum Denoising Software

Beyond optimized scanning techniques and streak removal, it is also possible to minimize the overall noise left in the final reconstructed image. Toshiba's *Quantum Denoising Software (QDS)* is an adaptive noise reduction filter that

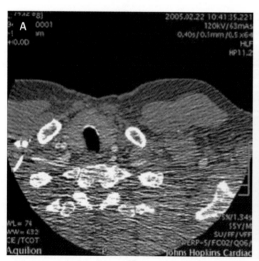 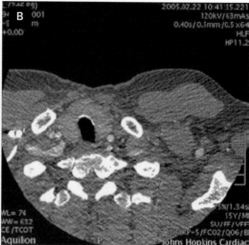

Figure 8.16. Effect of Boost^{3D} on streaks from low photon count. **A:** Typical streaks through the shoulder region. B: The same dataset reconstructed with Boost^{3D} with reduced streak artifacts.

works on reconstructed image data by preferentially smoothing areas of uniform density while preserving the edge information in the image. The algorithm uses locally sampled edge information within the image to blend together variable strength smoothing and sharpening filters. In areas of uniform density with few edges, the algorithm smoothes the image and reduces the noise; in areas with edges, such as near tissue boundaries and other complex structures, the algorithm enhances the image. QDS works in both two and three dimensions and can drastically reduce image noise, allowing a corresponding savings in patient dose. With QDS, it is possible to reduce the mAs by as much as 50% without compromising image quality. QDS works in conjunction with the [SURE]Exposure3D software to adjust the mAs based on the expected noise reduction from the adaptive filter. In this way, patient dose reduction is totally integrated in the Aquilion console software.

[SURE]Cardio Prospective

A considerable amount of attention has been focused on dose reduction in coronary CT imaging, which has traditionally been one of the higher dose CT exams. Although some approaches concentrate on dose reduction via step and shoot acquisitions, Toshiba recognized the inherent limitations of such an approach when the detector coverage is less than the entire heart. A primary limitation is that data can only be acquired every other heart beat, resulting in long study times. Early studies with this approach have shown significant contrast differences between acquisitions as well as discontinuities and non-diagnostic segments in nearly a quarter of the patients imaged. Another major limitation of the step and shoot approach is that it is limited to heart rates less than 65 bpm.

Toshiba's [SURE]*Cardio Prospective* software avoids the image quality issues associated with acquiring data every other heart beat by improving current helical dose modulation techniques and turning the x-rays completely off during portions of the cardiac cycle. With this approach, it is possible to lower the dose significantly more than by simply reducing the mA during systole. This is attributable to the fact

that the x-rays can be turned completely off much faster than they can be reduced to 10-15% of the max power. When the mA is simply reduced, there are ramp up and ramp down times that contribute to overall patient dose. In this way, [SURE]Cardio Prospective can reduce the patient dose by up to 80% compared with a non-modulated exam taken with the same mA and tube voltage (kVp) techniques.

Perhaps the greatest advantage to the [SURE]Cardio Prospective approach is the flexibility afforded with different patient heart rates. For patients with slow, steady heart rates, the scan can be acquired at very low doses in about 6 s. For faster heart rates, it is still possible to use [SURE]Cardio's clinically validated, adaptive segmented reconstruction to optimize the exams temporal resolution. Furthermore, if the patient's heart rate becomes erratic during the scan, [SURE]Cardio Prospective will automatically return to conventional, retrospective helical acquisition ensuring a diagnostic study. This high level of flexibility brings predictability and consistency to the cardiac acquisition. As opposed to the step-and-shoot approach, with this approach is possible to know a priori how long the exam will take based on the patient's heart rate and anatomy and, therefore, it is possible to know exactly how much contrast will be needed. These advantages to the [SURE]Cardio Prospective approach ensure that a diagnostic exam is acquired every time.

Variable Helical Pitch

There are several common CT exams that evaluate contrast flow in neighboring anatomy. The chest pain triage exam looks at the coronary arteries, the pulmonary arteries, and the thoracic and abdominal aorta. This sort of exam is typically administered with a single contrast injection and a low-pitch, ECG-gated acquisition. A critical limitation to this approach is that the pitch required for the ECG-gated acquisition is very low and contributes to a very high patient x-ray dose for these exams. However, although it is necessary to gate the exam for the coronary anatomy, the remaining abdominal aorta portion does not need to be gated. Similarly, other exams will image the coronaries and follow-up with a study of the renal vasculature or the peripheral vasculature. Typically, these exams require multiple contrast injections as well as multiple helical acquisitions to image the targeted anatomy. In both of these cases, a significant reduction of x-ray dose and iodinated contrast dose could be realized if the scanner could combine the multiple studies into a single acquisition without resorting to unnecessary ECG-gating of noncardiac anatomy.

To achieve this vision, Toshiba developed its *variable Helical Pitch (vHP)* acquisition mode. vHP allows the user to prescribe an exam that changes the helical pitch on the fly within a single acquisition. For example, the scanner will acquire at an ECG-gated pitch through the coronaries and then speed up the table to a standard pitch for the abdominal aorta, the renal vasculature, or even continue all the way down through the peripheral vasculature in the legs without stopping the table or reinjecting the contrast material. By adapting the reconstruction to the changing speed of the table, the entire volume can be reconstructed as a single study or broken up into its constituent pieces. This way, these high x-ray dose exams that use significant amounts of contrast agent and take multiple acquisitions can be accomplished with only one injection of contrast and at a lower dose.

The primary dose savings with vHP scanning comes from not gating portions of the exam that do not need to be gated. A typical pitch used for cardiac gating is 0.2, which means that the scanner overlaps by 80% for every rotation. This is necessary to image a rapidly moving heart, but creates an unnecessarily high dose acquisition in the abdomen. By transitioning to a standard pitch once the coronaries are done, the dose to the abdomen can be reduced by nearly 70%.

For multiple acquisition exams, such as a coronary exam followed by a renal study or a peripheral run-off, the dose savings come from not overlapping the volumes and requiring only one set of helical over-ranging instead of two. To allow two exams of neighboring anatomy to be registered properly, the two volumes often overlap somewhat to ensure that all the anatomy is covered. For all helical exams, there is an amount of over-ranging, i.e., the run-in and run-out portions of the exam that allow the edges of the volume to be reconstructed. The amount of over-ranging is fixed based on the pitch. Therefore, the percent contribution of over-ranging to the total exam dose goes up as the scan length goes down. Two short exams have twice the amount of over-ranging as with a single long exam. Therefore, by acquiring the entire anatomy in a single variable helical pitch run, the volume overlap and extra over-ranging can be avoided, saving dose to the patient.

Beyond the 64-Slice Scanner

Multiple-slice CT acquisition revolutionized the way patients are imaged and data are analyzed. The ability to view an entire volume with thin slices opened the door to a world of new diagnostic tasks for CT. However, to cover entire organs, MDCT requires helical scanning. Because of the limited coverage of MDCT, the volumes acquired for whole organ motion and perfusion studies are not temporally uniform because each portion of the volume is acquired at different moments in time.

The next revolution in CT technology comes with the ability to acquire an entire organ with isotropic resolution in a single gantry rotation.

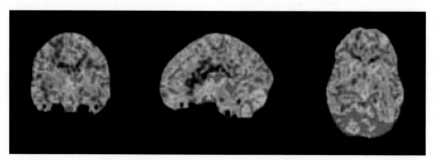

Figure 8.17. Whole-brain perfusion in the coronal, sagittal, and coronal planes. Taken from a single dynamically acquired dataset during contrast infusion (Aquillion ONE dynamic volume CT–320-row MDCT scanner).

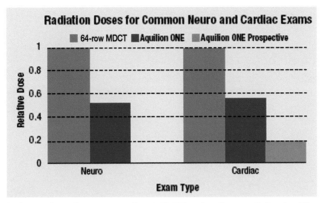

Figure 8.18. Graph of relative doses between 64-slice MDCT technology and the Aquilion ONE dynamic volume CT (320-row MDCT scanner).

This unique innovation enables dynamic volume scanning, allowing physicians to visualize dynamic flow, dynamic motion, and entire anatomical volumes at a single moment in time. Figure 8.17 shows a dynamically acquired neuro dataset on the Aquilion ONE (320 row × 0.5 mm). From a single dynamic dataset, it is possible to evaluate the cerebral vessels in arterial phase, in venous phase, in a dynamic subtraction cine loop, and also determine perfusion metrics such as cerebral blood flow, cerebral blood volume, and mean transit time.

Beyond the clinical advantages that dynamic volume CT affords, it can also significantly reduce the x-ray dose to the patient. With 16 cm of z-axis coverage using 320 rows of 0.5 mm detector elements, an entire coronary study can be acquired in a single 350-ms rotation of the gantry. By eliminating the need for the low helical pitch required for multislice cardiac imaging, the dose can be reduced by as much as 80% compared to similar multislice mA and kV techniques. Figure 8.18 shows the potential dose reduction using dynamic volume CT imaging using Aquilion ONE (320-row MDCT) scanner.

Summary

There are many factors that affect the x-ray dose to the patient. The Aquilion line of MDCT scanners is efficiently designed to create high-quality images at the lowest possible patient x-ray doses (Fig. 8.18). Software solutions such as Toshiba's

SURE Exposure3D, quantum denoising software, and Boost[3D] automatically adjust scan and reconstruction parameters to maximize image quality and reduce dose. Also, new scan modes such as SURE Cardio Prospective and variable helical pitch increase the utility and workflow of the scanner while driving the doses down even further. Finally, dynamic volume CT moves beyond multislice CT and produces complete volumes with a single rotation, creating the best images at the lowest doses yet. Toshiba Medical Systems designs the ALARA principle into every Aquilion CT scanner delivering high quality diagnostic images while minimizing patient dose.

Conclusions

In this chapter, various strategies developed by major CT manufacturers were discussed. Adopting these strategies and customizing CT protocols and implementing in day-to-day practice leading to reduction in radiation dose ultimately fall in the hands of the CT end users. Beside all these built-in features, a large potential for dose saving lies in the optimal and dose-efficient design of clinical applications. Users need to understand some basic details of dose and strategies to save dose in clinical routine. To fully exploit the benefits of CT imaging, all of us involved in CT imaging should adopt and implement various strategies no matter how small they are to minimize the harmful effects of radiation dose.

9

Hybrid Imaging Systems: PET-CT and SPECT-CT

Imaging modalities commonly are differentiated as functional or anatomical in nature. However, both categories of information are complimentary for integration of data for diagnosis, planning, performance, and evaluation of cancer therapy. Interpretation of nuclear medicine functional images is improved when they are coregistered with anatomical images. The explosive growth of dual modalities, such as positron emission tomography/computed tomography (PET-CT) and single-photon emission computed tomography/computed tomography (SPECT-CT), attests to the value of fusing form and function. It has been just less than a decade (the first commercial PET-CT scanners were introduced in 2001 in the United States) and already an estimated >1.5 million PET-CT scans per year were performed in 2007. Now most clinical PET studies are performed as PET-CT scans and nearly all PET scanners sold currently are PET-CT scanners, not dedicated PET devices. Similar trends are emerging with SPECT-CT imaging. Dual-modality scanners or hybrid scanners such as PET-CT or SPECT-CT became practical only after the introduction of multiple-row detector CT (MDCT).

Positron Emission Tomography/Computed Tomography

The advantages of combining a CT scanner with a PET scanner are multiple. Both the PET and the CT scans are fully registered and if performed with correct technique without patient motion, will allow the online fusion of two sets of volumetric images of different types. PET provides functional images of radiopharmaceutical distributions. CT provides anatomical images used for localizing radiopharmaceutical update and that also supply attenuation maps, which allow for attenuation correction to be performed, allowing for more quantitatively accurate PET reconstructions. CT also provides intrinsically useful anatomical information, which is of clear diagnostic value, even if the CT is not performed at the absolutely highest diagnostic performance levels.

The advantages of using a CT scanner with a PET scanner in the so-called hybrid imaging systems are that the CT data improves anatomical landmarks for the localization of radiotracer uptake. This is attributable to high photon flux, which improves accuracy and reduced noise levels of attenuation measurements and much greater quality images than those from radionuclide sources. CT also provides high spatial resolution images that can generate highly accurate localization maps and also accurate attenuation correction maps.

Because the average CT energy is in the range of less than 100 keV and the PET energy is in the range of 511 keV, there is little cross talk between the transmission and emission images. Of course, with all current PET systems, these images are obtained sequentially and not simultaneously. PET-CT scanners are designed so that the hybrid scanner is neither only PET nor only CT; it is truly a new imaging tool. It combines two major medical imaging technologies:

x-ray CT for anatomical imaging and attenuation corrections, with PET for functional imaging. The PET-CT scanner can operate as a single or a dual modality system, which can be used to acquire only CT scans, only PET scans, or PET-CT scans.

Figure 9.1 shows a schematic drawing of a typical PET-CT scanner. The CT gantry is positioned parallel to the PET gantry. Both the CT gantry and the PET gantry are assembled such that they are positioned in line so that the two components, the PET scanner and CT scanner, can relatively easily be separated to allow for performing repairs or maintenance services on individual scanners, and in line so that the scanners image the same portion of each patient if the table is properly incremented between the devices. The fact that the devices are next to one another, albeit closely integrated, means that each component, the CT and the PET, can advance at its own rate in terms of improvements in technology.

In practice, many manufacturers offer several choices of CT scanner performance (e.g., slice number, rotational speed, number of x-ray tubes) that can be paired with the same (or varying) PET scanner performance characteristics.

Thus, very high slice number (such as 64-slice MDCT) scanners for CT scanning may be most appropriate for the CT component of PET-CT scanners used in the management of cardiovascular disease, where CTA may be a part of the PET-CT, whereas lower CT slice numbers (4- or 16-slice MDCT) and slower rotational speeds may be quite adequate for most oncological applications.

Because the PET and the CT scanners adjoin one another closely but do not perform the PET scan and the CT scan at the same time (or the same place) on the patient, it is critical they be aligned carefully. Further, to have the patient imaged at the same exact point with both modalities, in all current systems, the imaging table must be advanced between the PET and the CT a distance equal to the separation between the gantries to image the same region of the patient. Thus, the table must be "in line" and the PET and CT components of the scanner must be aligned properly in multiple dimensions.

An initial challenge in the development of clinical PET-CT scanners was the stability of the patient table. When the table was extended such that the head of the table is positioned all the

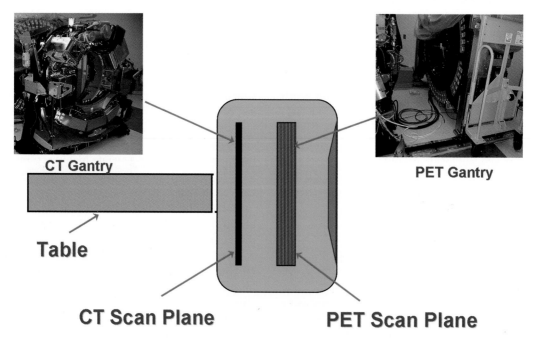

Figure 9.1. Schematic diagram of CT and PET gantry in a PET-CT scanner. The diagram shows the CT gantry followed by the PET gantry.

way inside the PET gantry, even a minimal flexion or bending of the table could result in a significant error in the image fusion processes as the patient would be more posterior on the table which has been flexed posteriorly. Hence, the stability of the patient table when positioned with maximum extension was an initial challenge in the design of these systems.

In some early designs, if the table was cantilevered over varying distances, especially with heavy patients, the patient weight would force the table downward if extended further. Thus, there could be a misregistration, with the patient more posterior on the PET image than the CT. Manufacturers avoid this in a variety of ways in current models. However, installation of a PET-CT scanner requires very careful attention to the floor position so that the floor is flat where the scanner and bed are installed. Then, the table can move seamlessly and without deviation through the gantry.

A typical PET-CT protocol includes moving the patient first into the CT gantry to perform a CT scan of the region of interest (often much of the body) and then moving the patient further to the PET gantry to acquire PET scan of a similar region. For example, in one approach to PET scanning, during a whole body PET-CT scan, the patient is scanned with CT scanner from mid-ear to mid-thigh, and then the patient is positioned at different location/fields under PET gantry to acquire PET images. The distance of separation is equal to the separation between the CT and the PET image. In this section, characteristics particular to PET-CT, such as scan parameters and radiation dose for typical PET-CT protocols, quality control, and radiation shielding for PET-CT scanners and image artifacts unique to PET-CT, are discussed.

Scan Parameters for PET-CT. In a PET-CT scanner, CT and PET-CT scanners are assembled adjacently. The patient is transported through the x-ray CT gantry on a carefully aligned and controlled imaging table, where CT scan is generally performed initially and is followed by a PET scan. A typical PET-CT protocol is shown in Figure 9.2, wherein a patient initially undergoes a CT scan followed by a PET scan on the same area. The CT information is then used for two purposes. The first is to register the anatomical images obtained with CT fused with the PET

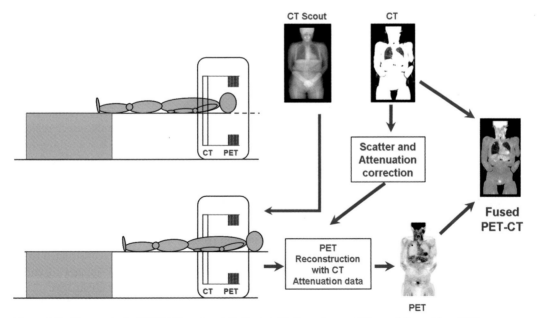

Figure 9.2. Shows a typical PET-CT protocol. Patients initially undergo a CT scan followed by a PET scan on the same region. The CT information is then used **(A)** to register anatomical images with PET images to display fused PET/CT images, and **(B)** CT information also is used for scatter or attenuation correction on PET scans prior to reconstruction PET images.

images to display as PET-CT images, and if a diagnostic quality CT is performed, for purposes of diagnosis. Second, the CT information is used for scatter correction or attenuation correction, which is used in the PET reconstruction. PET-CT images are displayed for the user's convenience both as an axial, coronal, sagittal, or a fused image and both PET and CT images can be displayed side by side and in any format the user wishes. This flexibility enables the clinicians to evaluate both the CT and also the PET images to make a suitable diagnosis.

Typical whole-body PET-CT scan parameters are as follows. This protocol is one used in many outpatient centers in which no intravenous contrast is administered. Such a protocol does not provide the highest-quality "diagnostic CT" examination, but it does provide important anatomic information which, when combined with PET, can result in highly accurate diagnoses. Normally a greater tube voltage (140 kVp) is used for better penetration through the thicker portion of the body such as the pelvis or shoulder, although this can vary by center and scanner. Some centers use 120-kVp x-rays because they are delivering a lower radiation dose and are often used in diagnostic CT. Also a weight-based tube current (mA) typically is used at some centers to minimize the radiation dose from CT. Other centers choose to use automated dose-adjustment algorithms provided by the manufacturers, although these are variable in their performance and, not uncommonly, have difficulty adequately penetrating the thicker portions of the shoulders or the region of the hips.

The typical mA settings for a whole-body PET-CT, along with other scan parameters, are shown in Table 9.1. Again, these parameters are not those used with fully diagnostic CT scans, which vary greatly depending on the part of the body being evaluated. It is certainly possible to combine a fully diagnostic CT scan with PET-CT, and this is done in some centers. One of the key technical factors is the selection of pitch. In PET-CT, because the CT image is reconstructed to match the PET slice thickness, a pitch greater than one is quite sufficient. However, generalizations about the CT chosen for PET are difficult, because a wide range of approaches can be

Table 9.1	Typical CT parameters for a whole-body PET-CT scan
Scan parameters	**Techniques**
Tube voltage	140 (to penetrate uniformly through thick portion of the body)
Tube current (weight based techniques)	80 mA for 150–200 lbs 60 mA for 100–150 lbs 40 mA for <100 lbs 120 mA for >200 lbs
CT gantry rotation time	1-s rotation
Pitch	1 to 1.5

applied in performing the CT as part of PET imaging, ranging from a relatively simple low-powered, high-pitched scan for attenuation correction and rudimentary lesion localization anatomically to a fully diagnostic thin-section CT angiography study (high-powered, low-pitch scans). One CT scan protocol increasingly does not fit all clinical situations.

The other key technical features for the PET-CT protocols are that a uniform large field of view is used for all patients and for all parts of the body, and the CT slices are reconstructed to thickness similar to PET slice thickness to facilitate fusion. More modern PET-CT scanners allow "zoomed" settings with reconstruction of smaller field of views (FOV) than the full possible FOV of the scanner. However, this is not commonly applied unless only select regional scans (such as head and neck scans) are done. Also, it is important to make sure that the CT reconstruction interval matches PET slice spacing for accurate image fusion. Even though the multiple-row detector CT (MDCT) can provide highest patient resolution, when the scanner is used in conjunction with the PET-CT scanners, the CT images are basically reconstructed to the slice thicknesses of the PET images to enable proper fusion of the PET and CT images.

However, newer scanners and software allow for display of thinner, higher-resolution CT images than the PET, with fusion to interpolated PET images. Early PET-CT scanners only offered essentially the same CT and PET slice thickness. Typical PET-CT exams, such as a whole body, involve scanning of a subject from mid-ear region to mid-thigh. The CT scan typically takes from 15 to 35 s, whereas a PET scan of the same region can take from 15 to 30 min. Generally, to achieve the most accurate quantitative PET imaging results, no contrast is used for the CT part during PET-CT scan because introduction of contrast can affect attenuation maps. Typically shallow breathing is allowed to match the breathing nature during the PET scans. Although MDCT scanner have faster gantry rotation time (less than 0.4 s), still the scan time chosen during PET-CT protocol can be lengthened slightly greater than half a second is used to minimize motion artifacts, though this remains somewhat unproven and a slower CT scan can degrade CT quality, especially if free tidal breathing is allowed. The CT axial scans are reconstructed so as to match the PET section for accurate attenuation correction.

Radiation Dose. The radiation dose from CT scan portion in the PET-CT scanner needs careful evaluation, and efforts are to be taken to reduce the overall radiation dose to the patient. A patient undergoing PET-CT receives radiation dose from both the PET and CT scanners. Because the CT part of PET-CT does not invariably require the very highest diagnostic image quality, the technical factors can be set such that the radiation dose is according to the "as low as reasonably achievable" (ALARA) principle. With the typical PET-CT scan parameters for a whole body PET-CT scan, such as 140 kVp, 80 mA (average size patient) and pitch of 1.5 can yield a CT dose 10 mSv (5–15 mSv range). This is in addition to a PET dose of approximately 15 mSv (10–20 mSv depending on the quantity of injected isotope). PET-CT, resulting in approximately 25 mSv (15-35 mSv range) per PET-CT scan, is considered a high-dose procedure. Table 9.2 shows effective dose values for typical diagnostic CT scans along with the PET-CT scans. Although the CT doses from the described non-contrast PET-CT protocol are lower than a typical diagnostic CT, CT doses still can contribute to nearly 40% of the PET-CT doses.

Examining the results of the radiation doses in an oncologic FDG PET-CT protocol, the CT

Table 9.2	Typical effective dose values with PET-CT and SPECT-CT in comparison with other standard diagnostic CT scans

CT procedure	Effective dose, mSv
Head CT	1–2
Chest CT	5–7
Abdomen and pelvis CT	8–11
PET-CT[a]	5–15
SPECT-CT[b]	2–5

[a] PET-CT scan includes scanning from mid-ear to mid-thigh on an average size adult. The effective dose values listed above is for the CT scan only. The effective dose for the PET scan with 25 mCi FDG is approximately 15 mCi. Therefore, for a typical PET-CT scan, the effective dose can range from 20 to 40 mSv.
[b] SPECT-CT scan includes scanning in a step and shoot mode with low tube current (2.5 mA), half-scan (acquisition time of 14 s per slice) and with fixed beam collimation of 10-mm full rotation mode scanning mid-ear to mid-thigh on an average size adult. CT contributes additional 6–12% of dose to patients undergoing SPECT-CT compared with SPECT only.

dose accounted for nearly 60% of PET dose for a protocol that included base of the skull to mid-thigh and 61% from the vertex of skull to mid-thigh and 65% from head to toe scan. The CT dose as percentage of total PET-CT dose was typically 37% for a skull base to mid-thigh protocol, 38% vertex of skull to mid-thigh protocol. and nearly 40% for head to toe protocol (please see "Suggested Readings" section for more information). The CT doses in PET-CT are typically lower than the typical diagnostic CT of the same region because of the lower tube current and the higher pitch values. Overall, the effective doses from CT range from 5–15 mSv and account for approximately 40% of the total effective dose during PET-CT.

Quality Control and Shielding Requirements. Although the quality control for CT scanners is discussed in chapter 11, there are some quality control procedures unique to integrated PET-CT systems. Most notably, the alignment of the PET and CT scanners must be correct. There are a variety of phantom systems that allow for visualization of both radioactive and radio-opaque spheres. The alignment provides assurance that the spheres are properly aligned when imaged by both PET and by CT.

These need to be checked periodically, but most critically, if there is any manipulation of the scanners or the bed as a part of camera service.

Although radiation shielding for CT scanners is discussed in chapter 11, there are some unique characteristics to be considered while shielding a PET-CT facility. The most significant radiation is usually observed in the uptake room adjacent to the PET-CT scanner, where the patient may spend an hour or longer before the PET scan. The uptake room shielding requirements are commonly more stringent than those of the room housing the PET-CT scanner. In the PET-CT scanner room, the major contributor is scatter radiation from the CT scanner, whereas in the uptake room the patient acts as a radiation source

for which the room has to be well shielded to protect the adjacent areas.

Image Artifacts in PET-CT. There are unique image artifacts observed during PET-CT scans. Because CT and PET scans are obtained sequentially and not obtained simultaneously, misregistrations may occur as the result of patient motion and deep breathing. Lateral attenuation increases with arms at side. Lateral streak artifacts are common with reduced tube current. Best images are obtained with shallow breathing or with a near full expiratory breath hold for the CT scan. An example of a typical image artifact is shown in Figure 9.3. It is a classic respiratory motion artifact. In Figure 9.3A,

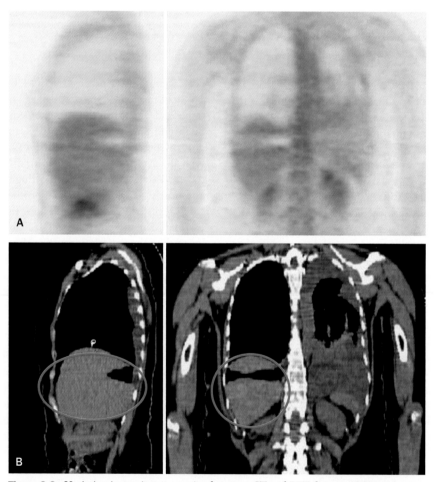

Figure 9.3. Variation in respiratory motion between CT and PET data acquisition can yield respiratory motion artifact on the PET image. **A:** PET image shows the dome of the liver sliced. **B:** CT scan indicates partially detached liver as the result of respiratory motion.

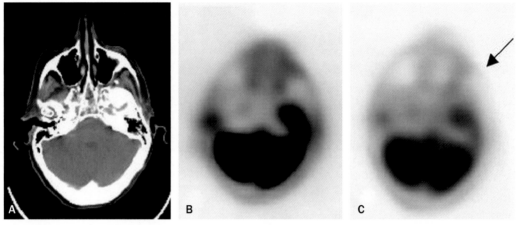

Figure 9.4. As shown, motion artifact can mislead diagnosis on PET scan. PET image with attenuation correction from CT data shows decreased tracer uptake in the left side of the face. Upon examining the CT (**A**), it appears the head was in a different direction during CT scan. This movement can lead to under correction of photon attenuation that results in decreased uptake on PET image (**C**); however, preattenuated corrected PET image (**B**) shows uniform uptake on the left side of the face this is attributable to under-correction of photon attenuation.

the PET image shows the dome of the liver sliced and upon examining the CT at the same position indicates a partially detached liver, which is due to motion artifact during the CT acquisition. This results in automatically demonstrating an artifact in the PET image also.

Figure 9.4 is an attenuated corrected PET image showing decreased tracer uptake in the left side of the face. This can be misdiagnosed; on looking at the CT scan image, one can see there is a head motion artifact and, because of this, there is an undercorrection of photon attenuation that resulted in a decreased facial uptake in the left side of the face.

Another classic artifact is a pacemaker artifact, which is visible on the attenuation-corrected PET and fusion images (Fig. 9.5). One can see a hot spot on the attenuated corrected PET image in the left anterior chest wall both on the PET and also on the CT image. However, on examining a nonattenuated corrected PET, the image appears to be normal. Therefore, it is important often to examine both the nonattenuated corrected PET image and the attenuated corrected PET image to eliminate some of these artifacts, which came from the CT attenuation. Similarly, in Figure 9.6, the artifact is caused by dense barium contrast. There is an increased

FDG uptake throughout the colon on attenuated corrected PET image. The corresponding CT slices show dense barium in the colon, which resulted in the error in the attenuation correction mass, which automatically translates to the increased FDG uptake. A nonattenuated corrected PET image shows normal bowel activity.

SPECT-CT

Around the same time when PET-CT scanners became commercially viable, similar efforts led to the introduction of SPECT-CT scanners. SPECT-CT systems have similar advantage as PET-CT and, furthermore, these systems allow patient-specific attenuation correction in both PET coincidence detection and single-photon emission tomography imaging. Unlike PET imaging, where the two photons always carry 511 keV, in SPECT imaging, the photon energy depends on the type of radioisotopes used. The most common isotope used is the technetium-99m (Tc-99m), with gamma rays carrying 140 keV of energy, whereas CT scans typically are performed at 120 or 140 kVp, with x-ray energies in the order of 40 to 60 keV. Unlike PET-CT, in SPECT-CT systems, the CT scan acquisition follows the SPECT scan. The residual

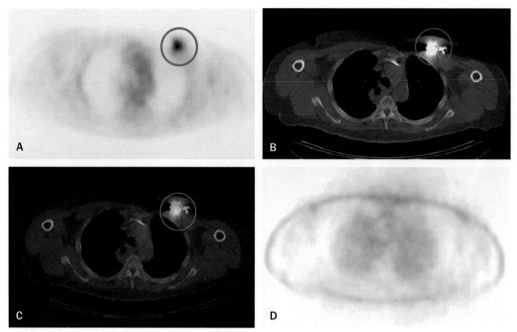

Figure 9.5. Pacemaker artifact that is visible on CT attenuation-corrected PET image in left anterior chest wall on PET, CT, and fused PET-CT image (**A–C**) but not visible on preattenuated corrected PET image (**D**).

isotope signals from patients undergoing CT scan soon after the SPECT study are of low flux and do not necessarily interfere with the x-ray flux of CT and therefore do not affect the CT images.

Unlike PET-CT, where all the CT systems are MDCT scanners, SPECT-CT systems can be broadly grouped into two distinct groups based on the type of CT systems. First, SPECT-CT systems with MDCT scanner positioned behind the SPECT system (Fig. 9.7), which has the capability to yield either 4, 6, 16, or 64 slices per gantry rotation. In these systems, similar to PET-CT, all range of CT protocols is available. The SPECT and MDCT scanner can be used independently or jointly as hybrid scanners. Full range of diagnostic quality CT imaging is possible on these systems, although in most hybrid scanning protocols, the CT scans are performed at lower techniques so as to yield lower radiation dose to patient yet provide sufficient x-ray photons for attenuation corrections for the SPECT images. Typical scan protocols on these systems include a scout scan or topograph survey scan on the MDCT scanner, followed immediately by the SPECT scan and later by a MDCT scan. The scout-scan assists in coregistering SPECT and

CT images. Often, the CT scan data are only used for attenuation correction and not for image fusion. In other cases, both attenuation correction and fusion of SPECT images with CT images are performed. Also, because these systems have a regular MDCT scanner, one has the option to perform additional CT scans, such as calcium scoring or CT angiography, all during a single visit.

On the other hand, the second group of SPECT-CT system is distinctly different in terms of the CT scanner. In these systems, a dedicated CT scanner is not a spiral CT scanner but a simple conventional "step-and-shoot" type of CT system with low-power x-ray tube and longer scan-time. In these systems, the CT scanner yields either a single-slice CT image of 10-mm slice thickness for each gantry rotation or as in recently available SPECT-CT system yields four images of 5-mm slice thickness (4 × 5 mm), mimicking a MDCT scanner but with low power and longer scan time. In these systems, the CT scanners are positioned between the SPECT camera and SPECT gantry (Fig. 9.8). These systems appear to play an intermediate role between nuclear medicine only system at one end of the

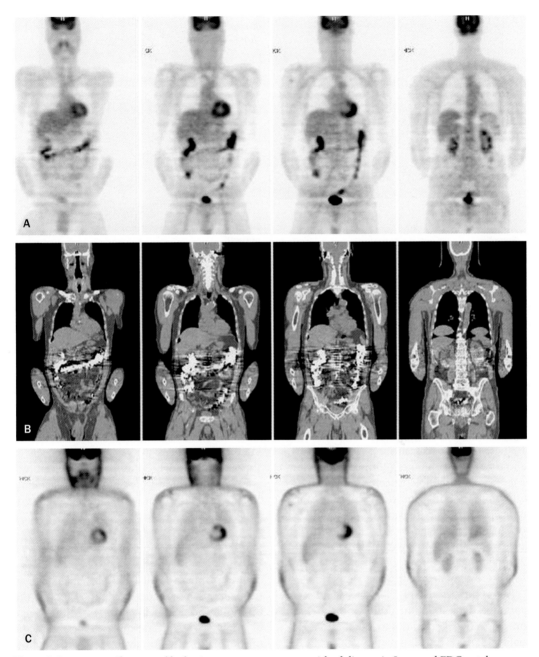

Figure 9.6. Image artifact caused by barium contrast agent can mislead diagnosis. Increased FDG uptake throughout colon on CT attenuated corrected PET image (**A**) caused by the accumulation of barium contrast agent in the colon. **B:** Pre-attenuated PET image shows normal bowel activity.

spectrum and full diagnostic quality hybrid imaging system at the other end of the spectrum.

In these systems, the x-ray tube and a set of detectors are mounted on opposite sides of the gamma camera gantry. The scan protocol includes SPECT scan followed by the CT scan. The CT scanner has a fixed anode oil-cooled x-ray tube operated at 140 kVp and tube current of 2.5 mA (maximum) with detector capability to provide a single 10-mm slice thickness or

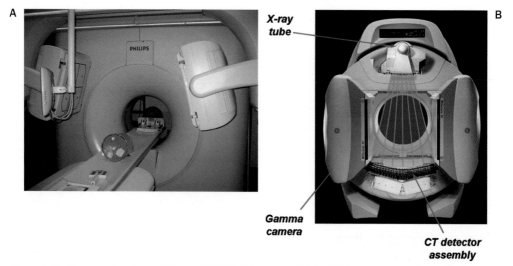

Figure 9.7. Photographs of two different SPECT-CT systems: **(A)** SPECT-CT system with 16 slice MDCT scanner (Precedence SPECT-CT, Philips Medical Systems) and **(B)** SPECT-CT system with a dedicated CT scanner (Infinia-Hawkeye, GE Healthcare, Waukesha, WI)

4 × 5 mm (20-mm coverage) slices per gantry rotation. The x-ray tube and detector rotate synchronously at a speed of either 26 s for full gantry rotation or 13 s for half gantry rotation acquisition. The total scan time to cover a region of 30 cm (similar to scan range for Chest CT) can range from 7 minutes (20-mm beam width or 4 × 5 mm multiple-detector configuration) to 14 min (10-mm beam width with single slice configuration). The radiation dose from CT portion of a whole-body SPECT-CT scan can range from 2 to 5 mSv, accounting for nearly 6–12% additional dose for those undergoing SPECT-CT compared with SPECT only scans.

The two types of SPECT-CT systems often evoke questions about the utility of the CT systems. First, how critical it is to have a diagnostic quality MDCT scanner in line with a SPECT scanner when the CT scanner is used only for limited period and therefore raises the question regarding the use of expensive diagnostic CT scanners. However, these scanners provide a wide range of applications that can be used, and additional scans can be completed during a single visit. Second, regarding SPECT-CT system using dedicated CT scanner (low-power, longer scan time, nonhelical), how useful are these systems because they have limited application

capability and require separate visit for diagnostic quality CT scans. However, these systems appear to satisfy niche markets that are expecting lower cost hybrid SPECT-CT systems.

Although there are two distinct types of SPECT-CT systems available, commercially it appears increasingly that most manufacturers are moving toward systems with standard MDCT scanners that can provide wide range of applications on these hybrid systems.

Conclusion

Hybrid scanners or dual-modality imaging systems are fast becoming the optimal tool in the diagnosis and treatment of cancer. A wide range of studies across diverse disease types has demonstrated consistent advantages with hybrid scanners as compared with PET, SPECT, or CT alone. Precise localization of pathology can drastically change the patient's diagnosis, management, and prognosis. In fact, PET-CT alone has the potential to become the ultimate imaging and treatment-planning device for cancer patients. The proper use of CT scanners to address the clinical question at a reasonable radiation dose remains in evolution and the approach may differ markedly in terms of CT

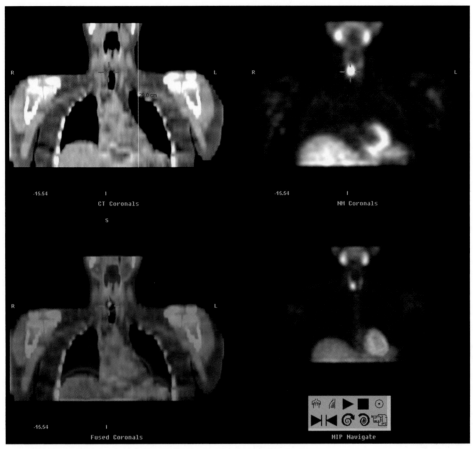

Figure 9.8. Images from a SPECT-CT system with dedicated CT scanner.

technique depending of the diagnostic question raised. Thus, one CT protocol does not fit all, but must be tailored to the specific patient for best outcomes. Overall, hybrid imaging has the potential to be used extensively in the future in solving increasingly complex clinical questions related to diagnosis and monitoring therapeutic outcomes.

10

Dual-Source CT and 320-Slice MDCT and Special Applications: CT Fluoroscopy and CT Perfusion

The fundamentals of multiple row detector computed tomography (MDCT) scanners and various detector designs were discussed in Chapter 3. Two major developments in recent years have been the introduction of dual-source CT (DSCT) and 256- to 320-row MDCT scanners, each of which have unique advantages and have created many new clinical applications. In addition, applications such as CT fluoroscopy and CT perfusion are discussed in this chapter.

Dual-Source CT

The temporal resolution has been one of the challenges in MDCT, even with the fastest rotating scanners, with scan time of 0.33 s (330 ms). Even with partial scans, the best temporal resolution that can achieved is approximately 165–185 ms, with a desired temporal resolution of less than 100 ms still elusive. A temporal resolution less than 100 ms can be achieved with multiple-segmented reconstruction but only after a trade-off of spatial resolution. The drive toward dual-source CT has been to further improve temporal resolution. In fact DSCT has been designed primarily to increase the temporal resolution of the MDCT system. The DSCT system is similar to 64-slice MDCT scanner but is equipped with two x-ray tubes and two corresponding detectors mounted in perpendicular orientation inside the CT gantry (Fig. 10.1).

The first detector set and x-ray tube is similar to single x-ray tube 64-slice MDCT scanner with scan field of view of 50 cm in diameter, whereas the second detector set is smaller in size with the

field of view of only 26 cm in diameter as the result of space limitations inside the gantry (Fig. 10.2). With two x-ray tubes and two detectors, the scanned data required for the image reconstruction can be acquired in half the time needed by a single x-ray tube MDCT scanner. At gantry rotation speed of 0.33 s, the temporal resolution of the DSCT thus equals to a quarter of the rotation time, i.e., approximately 83 ms (Fig. 10.3).

As in the 64-slice MDCT scanner, the two sets of detectors consist of 40 detector rows, the 32 central rows having a 0.6-mm collimated slice width and the outer four rows on both sides having a 1.2-mm collimated slice width, yielding a maximum coverage of 28.8 mm in the longitudinal direction. Each detector, by using z-flying focal spot technique, combines two subsequent 32-slice readings with a 0.6-mm collimated slice width to one 64-slice projection with a sampling distance of 0.3 mm at isocenter. In this way, even though there are no 64 physical detector rows, it is still possible to obtain 64 slices with only 32 rows of detectors. Often DSCT is misunderstood and called a 128 slice-MDCT scanner and, in fact, DSCT is similar to 64-slice MDCT scanner except it has two x-ray tubes and scan data from two sets of detectors that are combined to improve temporal resolution.

As shown in Figure 10.2, the second detector set is smaller in size compared with the larger detector set, which limits using both tubes simultaneously for all types of imaging protocols. In fact, the primary motivation for the design of DSCT is to improve the temporal resolution, which is key for cardiac imaging. However, the

157

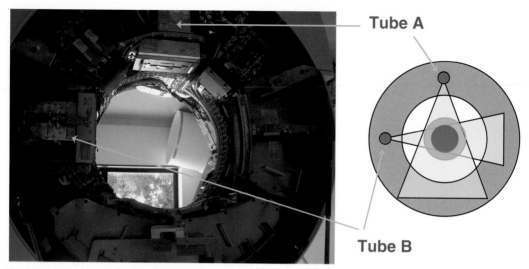

Figure 10.1. Photograph of DSCT (Definition, Siemens Medical Systems, Erlangen, Germany) gantry showing the two x-ray tubes and two detectors positioned orthogonally. Detector assembly B is smaller than detector assembly A and yields a smaller scan field of view than detector B.

DSCT scanner using only the x-ray tube with larger detector basically functions as a regular 64-slice single-source MDCT scanner. In addition to the advantage of using DSCT for cardiac imaging, the scanner also provides opportunities to explore new clinical applications. One such application is the potential to use DSCT for dual-energy scans. The dual-energy applications are not merely limited to providing images with x-ray attenuation differences but also provide entirely new ways to characterize functional and tissue characterizations during imaging.

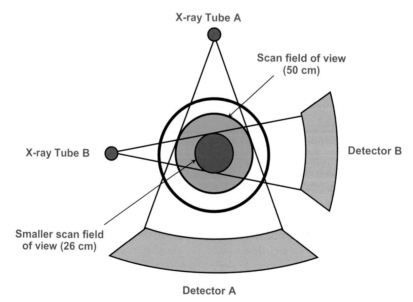

Figure 10.2. Schematic drawing of DSCT illustrating the available range of scan field of view. Detector A covers the entire scan field of view (50 cm in diameter) and is similar to 64-slice MDCT scanner. Detector B covers a smaller scan field of view (26 cm in diameter).

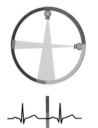 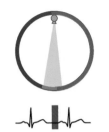

DSCT ~ 90 ms
90° Data Acquisition per tube
Scan time ~ 330 ms

64 Slice MDCT ~190 ms
180° Data Acquisition
Scan time ~ 330 ms

Figure 10.3. Temporal resolution that can be achieved with DSCT is compared with a 64-slice MDCT from the same manufacturer (Siemens Medical Systems, Erlangen, Germany) demonstrating improved temporal resolution with DSCT. Improvement in temporal resolution is achieved since by the use of scan data from one-fourth of the gantry rotation time from each of the x-ray tube is sufficient for image reconstruction.

Dual-energy CT applications become easier to achieve with DSCT scanners because each x-ray tube can be set at different tube voltages and therefore can obtain images at two different energies simultaneously. Many potential applications, such as separation of bones and iodine-filled vessels in CT angiography, characterization of kidney stones, and other tissues, are possible with DSCT. The full use of DSCT scanner with dual-energy CT applications can in principle add functional information in addition to the anatomical information usually obtained in a CT examination.

Dual-Energy CT Applications. Dual-energy computed tomography (DECT) applications have been of interest for a long time and are becoming a reality with the recent introduction of the DSCT scanner and with technologies capable of switching tube voltages and detectors designed in "sandwich"-type configurations to separate transmitted x-rays into different energies and other type of energy-discriminating detectors (photon-counting detectors). DECT applications have the potential to further push the CT technology from providing anatomical type of information to both anatomical and functional type of information with each examination.

Beyond 64-Slice: 256- and 320-Slice MDCT

With 64-slice MDCT scanners, the maximum anatomical coverage is confined to only 40 mm. This means that for cardiac imaging, it requires a minimum of three to five gantry rotations to cover the entire heart. This limits the width of coverage for continuous or cine type of imaging of the heart. Also, in cardiac imaging, to ensure a complete data set, a common procedure such as CT angiography is routinely performed with excessive tissue overlaps (low-pitch values with retrospective electrocardiogram-gated acquisition; see Chapter 6 for further details), resulting in a high radiation dose.

The desire to scan an entire organ such as the heart while still maintaining high spatial resolution led to the development of 256-row and, more recently, the 320-row MDCT scanner (Fig. 10.4). These scanners use a wide-area detector that is designed similar to the 64-row detector design, each approximately 0.5 mm × 256 or 0.5 mm × 320 mm with longitudinal coverage of 128 mm or 160 mm. With the use of large-area detector such as 320-row MDCT scanner, it is possible to cover the entire heart or head in a single gantry rotation. This provides new opportunities to perform not only anatomical coverage but also cine type imaging and capable of evaluating functional aspect in cardiac imaging.

In the 256-row MDCT scanner, the 256 row of detectors in the longitudinal direction can cover an area of 12.8 cm per gantry rotation at scanner isocenter and about 10 cm away from isocenter. Similarly, in the 320-slice MDCT scanner, the maximum coverage is 16 cm at the isocenter and about 12 cm away from the isocenter. The 320-row MDCT scanner allows continuous use of several collimation sets, including 320 × 0.5 mm for axial and helical type of data acquisition and 64 × 0.5 mm for axial and helical

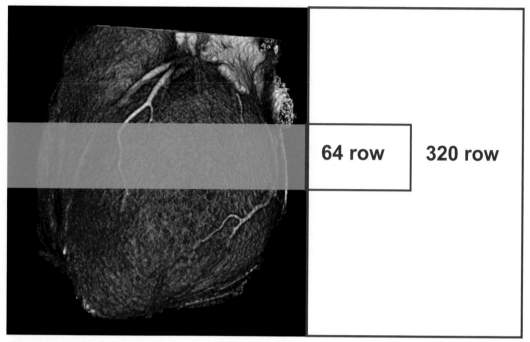

Figure 10.4. Diagram describing the scan coverage per single CT gantry rotation with a 320-row MDCT scanner compared with a 64-row MDCT scanner from the same manufacturer (Toshiba Medical Systems, Nasu, Japan). The maximum scan coverage with 320-row MDCT scanner is 160 mm at the scanner isocenter, with the ability to cover the entire heart in a single gantry rotation.

acquisition (similar to 64-slice MDCT scanner). Cone-beam artifacts caused by the nature of cone beam produced in 256- or 320-row MDCT scanners, can significantly diminish the advantage of large area detectors unless such artifacts are properly corrected or suitable type of image reconstruction algorithms specifically designed to handle cone-beams are used.

CT Fluoroscopy

CT fluoroscopy is similar to conventional CT, with the additional advantage of providing constant updates of the scanned data and therefore providing fluoroscopy type cross-sectional images. Unlike conventional fluoroscopy, the images are superimposition free and provide high contrast resolution images as the result of low scatter from narrow CT beam. CT fluoroscopy has been shown to be very useful in general interventions, in performing needle biopsy, drain placement, and many other procedures that require active intervention during the procedure.

To perform CT fluoroscopy, the CT facility needs to meet certain technical requirements, such as a CT table that can be readily moved in and out of CT gantry (i.e., a floating CT table) during the procedure in addition to a high-accuracy laser light marker with reference to the x-ray beam to aid in faster needle placement. Also needed are foot or manual switches to control individual scan acquisition, together with display monitors by side of the CT gantry so the operator can follow the procedure. Finally, real-time image reconstruction is needed with a delay between the activation of the foot switch and data acquisition that is as short as possible (normally <250 ms) and a delay between manual activation and display on the monitor that does not exceed 200 ms. Image reconstruction is achieved by using partial scan data and also by temporarily overlapping data from the previous set of images. CT fluoroscopy using a MDCT scanner provides multiple images that more accurately reflect the position of the needle and its deviation from the target, which makes it easier to determine how the needle or table should be repositioned (Fig. 10.5).

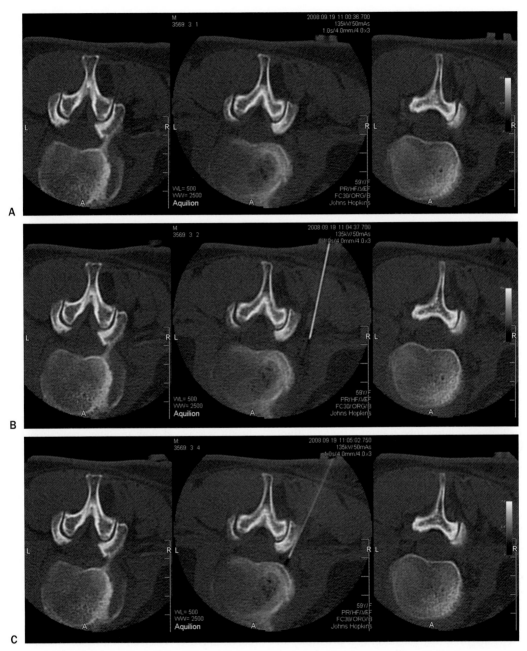

Figure 10.5. Images obtained during CT fluoroscopy procedure performed on a 64-slice MDCT scanner are shown. Three 4-mm thick images are displayed during each CT fluoroscopy exposure. Multiple thin images show more accurately the needle position with respect to the target of interest and allow user to easily manipulate the needle in the right direction. **A:** Target location is identified before the needle insertion. **B:** Needle position appears to be slightly away from the target, requires user to manipulate the needle insertion direction such that subsequent CT fluoroscopy images shows the needle is in the correct location.

Like conventional fluoroscopy, CT fluoroscopy provides image sequences over the same anatomical region and, therefore, the radiation dose from continuous exposure is a concern. Prolonged fluo-roscopy procedures have shown to have the potential to cause skin injuries as the result of a high cumulative radiation doses. Similarly with CT fluoroscopy, the continuous exposure to radiation can result in accumulation of large radiation dose to the same anatomical region, thereby increasing the potential for skin injuries.

As discussed previously, radiation-induced skin injuries are examples of deterministic effects, whereas other types of biological effect of radiation are considered stochastic effects. In routine CT, the primary concern is stochastic effects, but with CT fluoroscopy, in addition to stochastic effects, the deterministic effects also are of concern. Deterministic effects are defined as short-term effects and exhibit a threshold dose below which the effects are not visible and above which the effects increases linearly with dose and are visible within days to weeks. Examples include radiation-induced skin erythema, epilation, cataracts, and even death.

A cumulative dose greater than 2 Gy is considered the minimal threshold dose to cause certain types of radiation-induced skin injuries. Because CT fluoroscopy involves continuous radiation exposure to the same region, it uses a low milliampere setting, typically 10 to 50 mA, whereas conventional CT scanning typically uses 150 to 600 mA. However, the cumulative dose is impacted by the total scan time. Therefore, even with low tube current during CT fluoroscopy, the typical procedure time of 1–400 s can yield cumulative skin doses in the order of 2 Gy, which are sufficient to trigger the onset of radiation-induced injuries. Therefore, it is important to keep the exposure time as minimal as possible to minimize the risks for radiation-induced injuries. In fact, the protocol for CT fluoroscopy is set so that the system warns after certain time of continuous or intermittent exposures to avoid accumulating excessive dose.

Another problem with CT fluoroscopy is that the operator can receive a considerable dose as the result of scatter radiation and proximity to CT gantry. Those performing CT fluoroscopy should be familiar with the three pillars of radiation protection, namely time, distance, and shielding. Minimizing time by intermittent radiation exposure, standing further away from the CT gantry (scatter radiation decreases by the square of the distance from the x-ray source), and wearing protective shields (lead aprons, thyroid shields) reduces personal radiation exposure. Protective gloves (not the thin radiation

attenuating surgical gloves, Wagner LK, Mulhern OR, *Radiology* 1996;200:45–48) and special instrumentation such as a needle holder should be used to protect the hands of the person performing CT fluoroscopy.

CT fluoroscopy is a useful tool for more rapid and less risky performance of radiological interventions. With CT fluoroscopy, it is often convenient for patient who arrives for a CT scan to undergo interventions such as the needle biopsy at the same facility. Similar to conventional fluoroscopy, radiation doses to patient and operators have the potential to reach high levels and should be monitored carefully. With current MDCT scanners with scan times less than 0.5 s and rapid image reconstruction, the conventional step-and-shoot type of CT scanning are becoming quite viable and may be as fast as CT fluoroscopy.

CT Perfusion

CT perfusion studies have increasingly performed to evaluate cerebral perfusion in patients with acute stroke, evaluate cardiac functions in patients with chronic cerebrovascular diseases, and functional evaluation of various other organs. CT perfusion is a blood flow imaging application that analyzes the uptake of injected contrast to determine functional blood flow information about a region of interest. The region of interest (e.g., brain, heart, or liver) is scanned in the same position and at the same time intervals, as per the expected rate of change. Intravenous contrast is injected into the patient, and a region of interest is scanned repeatedly for a period of time. The CT number (measured in Hounsfield Units) enhancement is tracked for each voxel over time to produce tissue specific time-density curves. Measurements made from these time-density curves and user-selected input regions are used to create various parametric functional images.

Perfusion studies can be performed with magnetic resonance scanners, positron emission tomography, and single-photon emission computed tomography system, but they are hampered by limited availability, cost, and and/or patient tolerance. On the other hand, perfusion studies can be performed quickly with any standard spiral CT scanner but even more with MDCT scanners, and the perfusion maps can be

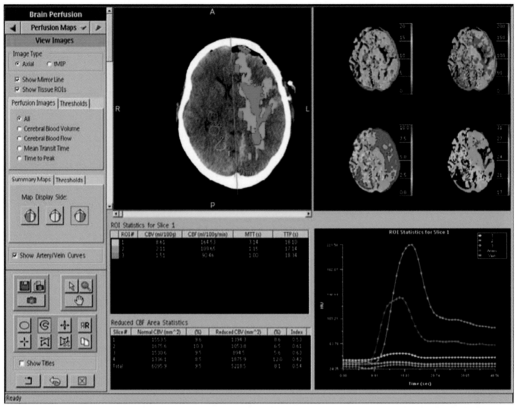

Figure 10.6. Typical CT perfusion maps showing CT image along with perfusion images showing blood flow, blood volume, and mean transit time images. In addition, CT perfusion software also displays blood flow statistics along with time-concentration curves for both artery and vein in the region of interest.

generated in a short time at a workstation equipped with the appropriate software. In fact, theoretical analysis of CT perfusion has appeared in literature back in 1980 and only after advent of spiral CT and more with MDCT has perfusion CT become practical.

The key parameters in CT perfusion are the measurement of blood flow, quantifying blood volume in the organ or region of interest, and mean transit time for the blood flow; these are calculated from the arterial, venous, and parenchymal time-density curves acquired by monitoring the first pass of contrast medium through a region of interest (Fig. 10.6). These parameters are evaluated by tracking the flow of contrast through the region of interest over time.

Because CT perfusion involves repeated scanning of the same regions, the radiation dose delivered to the same tissue region can be high and can exceed the minimum threshold dose required to cause radiation induced skin injuries.

Even with scan techniques such as 80 kVp, 200 mAs, 4 × 5-mm detector configurations and CT dose of 12 mGy, the total dose for 50 s of perfusion study can yield as much as 600 mGy (0.6 Gy). There is a need to optimize scan protocols during CT perfusion studies in order to minimize the potential for radiation induced skin injuries.

Conclusions

Advances in MDCT technologies, including DSCT and 256- or 320-row MDCT scanners, have led to many new applications, including CT fluoroscopy, CT perfusion, and dual-energy CT scanning. These applications have propelled MDCT technology from the current form of providing only anatomical information to more robust technology providing both anatomical and functional information paving path to even newer applications.

Quality Control and Radiation Protection

The description of various aspects of multiple-row detector computed tomography (MDCT) scanners, including scan parameters and radiation dose, were discussed in earlier chapters 7 and 8. Any discussion on MDCT is not complete without discussing quality control and radiation protection issues. It is even more crucial to understand the importance of radiation safety, especially in the era of increased regulations and concerns about radiation protection for those who work with or around radiation.

In addition, costs of the increasing number of CT procedures performed worldwide are adding onto the local, national, and global healthcare costs. To examine ways to reduce rapidly increasing healthcare costs, medical insurance reimbursement policies in the United States increasingly are examining the validity of new procedures and efforts are underway to tie the performance of the scanner with regard to image quality and radiation dose with the degree of reimbursement.

One path to examine the performance of image modality is through quality control programs. Increasing quality control requirements and accreditation programs that examine the quality of CT images with respect to performance are gaining widespread acceptance both from regulatory agencies and also from private insurance groups. Practical quality control programs to examine the performance of the MDCT scanners on a periodic basis are essential and are becoming mandatory. These programs should examine the overall performance of the system and also examine the radiation dose related to different protocols. Although there are no limits

regarding the radiation dose for various clinical protocols, efforts should be made to compare radiation doses, and it is beneficial for individual clinics to compare the radiation dose and image quality of their clinical protocols with the available reference dose levels. Any discussions on radiation dose are to be tied with image quality. Any efforts to lower radiation dose unilaterally without examining image quality defeats the overall purpose of reducing dose to patient because poor-quality images can result in repeat CT scans. Therefore, it is important to understand that the image quality and radiation dose are both intertwined in clinical protocols.

In this chapter, various aspects of quality control and radiation protection are discussed. Radiation safety with regard to patients was discussed in earlier chapters 7 and 8 on radiation dose and strategies on how to reduce dose. The emphasis of radiation protection is with regard to the protection of radiation workers and of general public. Radiation safety is further discussed under the purview of personnel radiation safety and the methods to monitor personal doses and the radiation shielding of the MDCT scanner room are given. A detailed description of all these topics can be found in most medical physics textbooks. Brief discussions of these topics, along with practical tips applicable to day-to-day practice, are provided in this chapter.

Quality Control

CT imaging continues to grow rapidly in the day-to-day clinical practice. With the introduction of

MDCT scanners, the number of CT procedures continues to grow at a rapid pace, often by double-digit percentages per year. This increase reflects the value that physicians are placing on the information provided by CT images and reflects the many new clinical applications in CT imaging that are the result of increasing quality and spatial resolution of images produced by MDCT scanners. Although there are no debates on the benefits of CT imaging, there is considerable debate regarding the potential risks of radiation from the CT exams. Therefore, it becomes essential to examine the performance of a CT scanner in terms of radiation dose and image quality by instituting appropriate quality control for MDCT scanners.

Quality control in general is defined as a program that periodically tests the performance of a modality such as MDCT scanner and compares its performance with some standard. If the scanner is performing suboptimally, then steps must be initiated to correct the problem to ensure proper quality patient care. Quality control is a subset of much larger quality assurance program. According to Papp's *Quality Management in the Imaging Sciences,* "Quality Assurance (QA) is an all-encompassing management program used to ensure excellence in healthcare through the systematic collection and evaluation of data. The primary objective of a QA program is the enhancement of patient care; this includes patient selection parameters and scheduling, management techniques, departmental policies and procedures, technical effectiveness and efficiency, in-service education, and image interpretation with timeliness of reports. The main emphasis of the program is on the human factors that can lead to variations in quality care. Quality assurance should not be confused with quality assessment, which is the measurement of the level of quality at some point in time with no effort to change or improve the level of care." On the other hand, "Quality Control is part of the QA assurance program that deals with techniques used in monitoring and maintenance of the technical elements of the systems that affect the quality of the image. Therefore quality control is the part of the QA program that deals with instrumentation and equipment." Under the masthead of quality control, the acceptance

test and periodic assessment of scanner performance play a key role in assuring availability of quality images from MDCT scanners.

Acceptance Test

The objective of acceptance testing is to assure that newly installed imaging equipment functions as designed, complies with regulatory standards, and produces high-quality images. Data collected during acceptance tests are useful in establishing baselines for future quality control testing. In addition, during the acceptance testing process, equipment set-up parameters can be customized to the preferences of the practice. Acceptance testing must be performed at the time of initial installation and whenever substantial modifications are made to the scanner, such as replacing the x-ray tube or detector array. The values measured must agree and fall within the tolerance levels of the manufacturer specifications and should serve as basis for all future quality control tests. According to certain regulatory agencies, acceptance tests are even mandatory. Whether or not the acceptance tests are mandatory, it is beneficial for any user to examine a newly installed scanner's performance and to establish initial performance of the scanner.

Various tests commonly performed as part of acceptance test include verifying CT number accuracy, homogeneity, radiation dose measurements, image noise, slice thickness, and low and high contrast resolution and spatial resolution (Table 11.1). These tests allow the user to verify the specifications of the scanner and also to establish baseline performance standards that can be used for comparing scanner performance in future.

Most MDCT manufacturers provide phantoms to evaluate the performance of their system (Fig. 11.1), and a few MDCT manufacturers provide phantoms containing different modules to examine various parameters along with automatic programs to analyze the performance of the scanner with preset criteria (Fig. 11.2).

In addition, it is important to examine or measure radiation dose by the use of standard phantoms (Fig. 11.3) and to compare it with the specifications of the scanners (±20–30%). All MDCT scanners are required to display the $CTDI_{vol}$ numbers. It is therefore, beneficial to compare the measured $CTDI_{vol}$ values with that

Table 11.1 Parameters or functions commonly recommended for acceptance testing, annual testing and periodic quality control testing in CT		
Parameter or function	**Acceptance and annual testing**	**Periodic quality control Testing**
Primary tests		
Dosimetry: CT dose index measurements	x	
CT number accuracy and homogeneity	x	x
Slice thickness	x	
Image quality	x	
Spatial (high-contrast) resolution	x	x
Low-contrast resolution	x	x
Image uniformity	x	x
Noise	x	x
Artifact evaluation	x	x
Image display – digital and hard copy	x	x
Secondary tests		
Accuracy of table position	x	
Light localizers	x	
Dose profiles	x	
Safety evaluation: visual inspection	x	
Scattered radiation measurements	x	
Patient dose for standard protocols	x	
Other tests as required by national or state or local regulations		

A subset of tests performed for acceptance and annual testing are recommended as part of periodic quality control program. Types, frequency and criteria's for periodic QC testing are normally recommended by qualified medical physicists.
Tests in accordance with the ACR CT accreditation program requirements and ACR technical standard for diagnostic medical physics performance monitoring of computed tomography equipment.

of the scanner display during the acceptance test. This provides confidence in using the radiation dose values displayed at the CT console in later times to estimate patient dose for any select protocol.

Periodic Quality Control

Periodic quality control tests are key to continuous assessment of CT performance. The type of test and frequency of quality control tests are to be established at the time of the acceptance test. Normally it is recommended that the qualified medical physicists determine the frequency of each test and identify who should perform each test based upon the facility and CT usage. The most common quality control test is the daily assessment of CT number accuracy. This is done by scanning a standard-size water phantom (provided by the CT manufacturer) to verify the accuracy of CT number for water, because all other

CT numbers displayed are normalized to voxel-containing water. On an annual basis, a subset of tests performed during the acceptance test are selected and performed for continuous evaluation of scanner performance (Table 11.1). Additional tests are performed depending on the regulatory requirements of the scanner location.

Among the number of resources available discussing the details of various quality control tests performed and recommended for MDCT scanners are the American Association of Physicists in Medicine (AAPM) task group report #39 and the American College of Radiology (ACR) technical standard for diagnostic medical physics performance monitoring of CT equipment and the ACR CT accreditation program guidelines.

Quality control programs independent of CT manufacturers are gaining ground in evaluating the performance of scanners. One such program gaining considerable attention is the ACR accreditation program for CT imaging. A specially

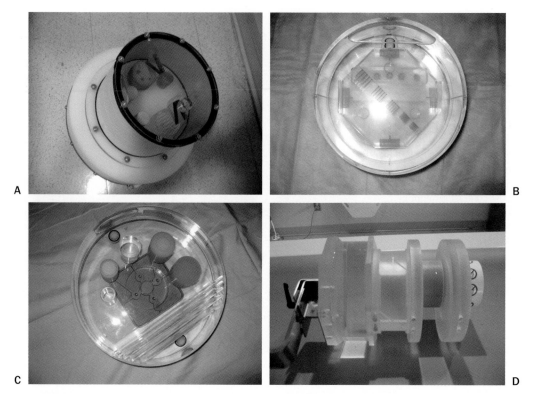

Figure 11.1. Photographs of quality control phantoms provided by different MDCT manufacturers a) Philips Medical Systems, b) GE Healthcare Systems, c) Toshiba Medical Systems and d) Siemens Medical Systems. Each phantom contains number of structures to evaluate performance of different imaging features.

designed CT phantom consists of four modules with specific test patterns to evaluate slice thickness, spatial resolution, contrast resolution, CT number evaluation, and image uniformity (Fig. 11.4). Although the accreditation for CT imaging is voluntary in the United States, certain private medical insurance agencies are requiring clients to be fully accredited before they can receive medical reimbursement. This trend appears to be gaining ground with rigorous quality control programs such as CT accreditation may soon become a requirement.

Radiation Safety

In terms of radiation safety to staff such as radiologists, cardiologists, technologists, and others, the personnel doses are normally minimal. Except during CT fluoroscopy, during all other CT scans, no one other than the patient is inside the scanning room. Because the scan rooms are shielded, the personnel doses are minimal.

However, during CT fluoroscopy the staff doses can be high depending on how close they are standing to the CT gantry. Therefore, it is required for all those who work with or around CT to wear radiation-monitoring devices to monitor personnel dose. Personnel doses should be within the limits established by respective regulatory agencies. For example, in the US, for radiation workers, the annual maximum permissible dose is 50 mSv (5 rem) (Table 11.2).

Radiation Shielding

The major purpose of shielding the MDCT scanner room is to protect individuals working with or near the MDCT scanner from radiation emitted by the scanner. With increasing x-ray beam widths, the shielding of a MDCT suite is critical in not only providing sufficient protection to the personnel working near or around the MDCT scanner but also to comply with the regulatory agencies requirements. Historically, imaging

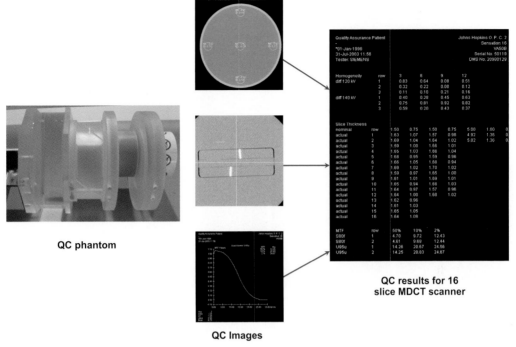

QC phantom

QC results for 16 slice MDCT scanner

QC Images

Figure 11.2. Photograph of a quality control phantom containing different modules to evaluate MDCT scanner performance. Also shown are the quality control images and results for a 16-slice MDCT scanner generated by an automated quality control program (from Siemens Medical Systems, Malvern, PA, with permission).

equipments were mainly housed in radiology departments, which has access to qualified medical physicists. However, the proliferation of MDCT scanners outside the realm of radiology departments and to physician offices often creates oversight regarding shielding and therefore requires careful evaluation of radiation protection in order to ensure safe use of MDCT scanner.

It suffices to say that the appropriate shielding estimation should be performed during the planning stages of acquiring a MDCT scanner and that appropriate shielding should be installed during the construction of the scanner room and verified after the installation of the MDCT scanner. The optimum time to verify installation of radiation shield is during the construction process before the

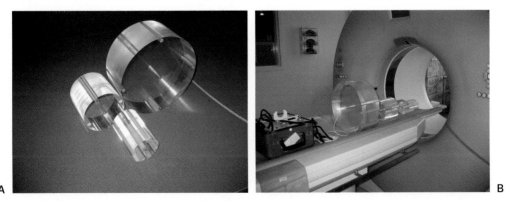

A   B

Figure 11.3. Photograph of standard CT dosimetry phantoms representing adult body (32 cm in diameter), adult head or pediatric body (16 cm diameter), and pediatric head (10 cm diameter) size. Also shown is the CT dose measurement setup.

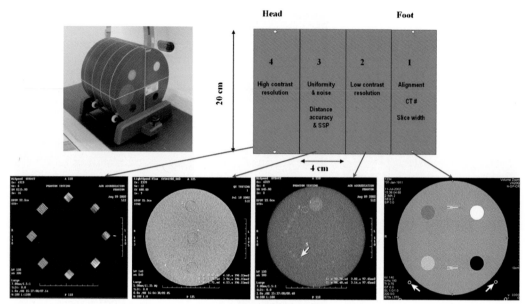

Figure 11.4. Photograph of the CT accreditation phantom from the American College of Radiology containing four modules to evaluate performance of different image features. Also shown are images corresponding to each of the four modules (from the American College of Radiology. Reston, VA, with permission).

completion of the scan room. This eliminates the more laborious measurement method of verifying shielding once the scan room is completed. The shielding process should be completed or reviewed with consultation with a qualified medical physicist to avoid any sort of interruption in MDCT service later due to regulatory lapses. Below is a brief discussion on how to shield a CT scanner.

Table 11.2 Annual maximum permissible radiation dose limits according to United States Nuclear Regulatory Commission[a]

Category		Maximum permissible dose limits	
		mSv[b]	rem
Radiation workers (occupational)	Whole body[c]	50	5
	Lens of the eye	150	15
	Skin or any extremity (hands, fee)	500	50
	Minor (<18 years old)	10% of adult limits	10% of adult limits
Pregnant woman, entire gestation (9 months)		5	0.5
General public (nonoccupational)	Whole body	1	0.1
	Lens of the eye	15	1.5
	Skin or any extremity (hands, feet)	50	5.0
Unrestricted area[d]		0.02 in any 1 h	0.002 in any 1 h

[a] US NRC Regulatory Guide 8.29 Revision 1, issue date February 1996.
[b] 1 mSv = 100 mrem.
[c] Limits are exclusive of natural background and any dose received for medical purposes by the individual.
[d] Dose to any area surrounding a radiation facility shall not exceed 0.02 mSv/h. This limit establishes criteria for estimating radiation shielding of CT facility.

The primary x-ray beam defined by the beam width (N*T) in a MDCT scanner, which is restricted by the beam collimation, is not the primary concern in shielding the CT scan room. It is the secondary, isotropic radiation, also known as scatter radiation, emitted from the patient, which is a primary concern and requires shielding to prevent it from reaching the adjacent areas. Therefore, for a MDCT scanner, all walls in the room are considered secondary barriers, because the detector array provides primary radiation barrier. The scattered radiation plots normally are provided by MDCT manufacturers as exposure lines from the isocenter of the gantry on a single slice basis for known mAs (Fig. 11.5a). The scatter radiation appears to spread out from the MDCT gantry in a butterfly pattern, because the MDCT gantry provides great attenuation at the scatter origin, i.e., the patient. The scatter radiation is highest on either side of the gantry and decreases significantly as one moves away from the gantry. According to inverse-square law (radiation dose inversely proportional to square of the distance from radiation source), the scatter radiation decreases by the square of the distance from the radiation source (patient in the CT gantry). In addition, the least amount of scatter is measured on the adjacent side of the CT gantry (Fig. 11.5b) because the gantry provides additional protection from scatter radiation.

Methods and technical information for the design of shielding for diagnostic x-ray rooms in general are found in NCRP report no. 147, entitled *Structural Shielding Design for Medical X-ray Imaging Facilities*, published in 2004. The amount of shielding required for a CT scanning room depends on several factors. The overarching principle in radiation protection and also in radiation shielding is the ALARA principle: to keep radiation dose "as low as reasonably achievable." The factors considered in estimating shielding requirements are the radiation exposure levels ("workload"), which are determined by the average number of patients planned to be scanned per week, the number of scans per patient, and the

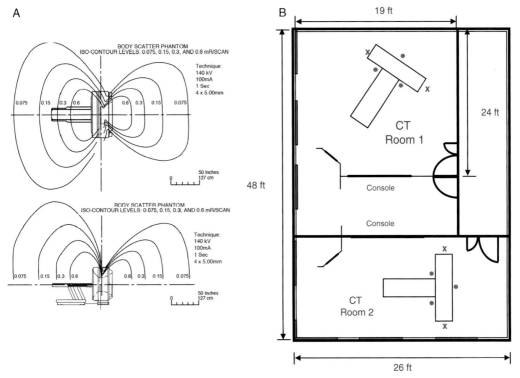

Figure 11.5. **A:** Scatter radiation plots demonstrating butterfly pattern around the CT gantry. **B:** Drawing of a CT suite indicating areas of high scatter (Red) and low scatter levels (Green)

average technique per scan. The "dimensions" of the scanner room and the "occupancy" of adjacent areas of the CT scanner and the "use factor" that determines the fraction of time radiation is incident on a particular wall are among the several other factors that are considered during estimating radiation shielding.

In addition, the regulatory limitations on the maximum allowed personnel exposures for both occupational (any one working with radiation) and nonoccupational (such as general public or non-radiation) workers may not exceed limits established by respective regulatory agencies. In the United States, these annual limits are 50 mSv (5 rem) for occupational workers and 1 mSv (0.1 rem) for nonoccupational personnel workers. In addition, the dose equivalent in an unrestricted area (public corridor or staircase or office spaces adjacent to CT scanner) may not exceed 0.02 mSv (2 mrem) in any hour.

For computing shielding requirements, normally "week" is used as unit of time. Therefore, for unrestricted areas such as general public areas the maximal allowance exposure limit is 0.02 mSv (2 mrem) per week and, for restricted areas, the maximum allowable exposure limit is 1 mSv (100 mrem) per week (Table 11.2). Shielding requirements are then computed based on occupancy around, below, and above the CT suite. Understanding the requirements set-forth by the regulatory agencies in respective state, country or jurisdiction is critical in order to protect any one working near or around MDCT scanner and also in minimizing any service disruptions during smooth operation of the MDCT scanner.

Scatter plots illustrate the need for variation in shielding, especially with increasing number of slices per gantry rotation implying larger x-ray beam width (16 × 0.625 = 10 mm,

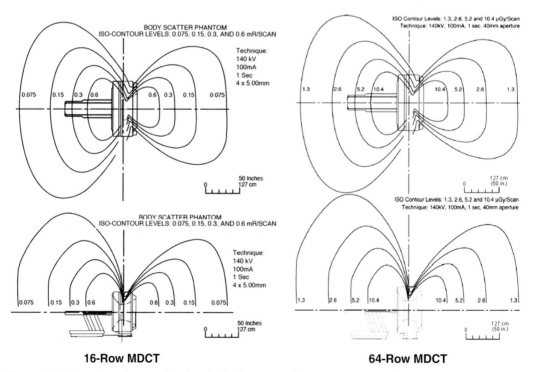

16-Row MDCT   **64-Row MDCT**

Figure 11.6. Drawings of scatter plots for a body phantom with a 16-row MDCT and a 64-row MDCT scanner from the same manufacturer. Even though the scatter plots appears similar for similar technique, the scatter radiation intensity is higher with 64-row MDCT because of larger beam width (20 mm on 16-row MDCT vs. 40 mm with 64-row MDCT). Therefore, depending on the size of the scanner room, occupancy of surrounding areas and many other factors, it may warrant additional shielding for 64-row MDCT compared with 16-row MDCT scanner (Printed with permission from GE Healthcare, Waukesha, WI).

64×0.625 mm $= 40$ mm to 320×0.5 mm $= 160$ mm) leading to increased scatter (Fig. 11.6). Normally in the United States, lead sheets of 1/16 inch (1.58 mm) thick attached to 5/8 inch (15.9 mm) gypsum board available in prefabricated form are used in radiation shielding construction. For a 16-slice MDCT scanner with typical workload, installed in a 6 m $\times$ 9 m room (20 ft $\times$ 30 ft), 1/16 inch of lead wall appears to be quite sufficient. However, with 64- or 320-slice MDCT scanners, shielding requirement appears to increase and may require 1/8 of an inch or greater depending on the occupancy adjacent to the MDCT scanner room. In the figure, the scatter intensity next to gantry shows marked differences in a 64-slice ($64 \times 0.625 = 40$ mm) compared with 16-slice (16×0.625 mm $= 10$ mm) MDCT scanner. Radiation shielding of MDCT scanners is normally performed by estimating reasonable workload on the planned scanner followed by overlaying the scatter plots provided by the manufacturer on the scaled drawings of the scanner room. This way, the required shielding to protect personnel in the adjacent areas is computed.

For a 64-slice MDCT scanner to be installed in a 6 m $\times$ 9 m room, and plans to perform predominantly cardiac CT scans of up to 20 patients per day and 5 days per week will require lead shielding as follows. On the basis of the regulatory requirement of less than 0.02 mSv per week

(1 mSv limit for nonoccupational worker for a year), the closest wall separating the CT scanner from office space located 3 m from the CT gantry requires a lead shielding of approximately 1.5 mm thickness. Details regarding shielding calculations and types of shielding materials can be found in NCRP report no. 147 entitled *Structural Shielding Design for Medical X-ray Imaging Facilities*, which was published in 2004. It is therefore generally recommended and required by certain regulatory agencies that the shielding process be completed or reviewed by a qualified medical physicist to provide suitable radiation protection to the adjacent areas surrounding the MDCT scanner and to avoid any sort of interruption in MDCT service later due to regulatory lapses.

Conclusions

Quality control and radiation protection are key aspects to be incorporated in to day-to-day practice in CT. Proper QC practice will enable smooth clinical operations and also enable to identify problems that could be corrected ahead of time and can reduce inconvenience that results due to untimely scanner downtime. Similarly, radiation protection is essential to ensure safety for all those who work with CT and also to comply with any standards and regulations set by various regulatory agencies.

Future Trends in MDCT

The future of multiple row detector computed tomography (MDCT) was easy to predict until now. From the time MDCT scanners (four-slice CT) became commercially available (Fig. 12.1), the discussion has been dominated by the so-called *slice-wars*, with manufacturers introducing scanners capable of yielding increasing numbers of CT slices. CT systems ranked based on the number of slices exhibited a kind of geometric progression, from single-slice to dual-slice with both nonhelical and helical single-detector CT (SDCT) scanner to 4-slice, 6-slice, 16-slice, 32-slice, 40 slice, 64-slice and, recently, 256- and 320-slice scanners (Fig. 12.1). Some MDCT scanners have as many physical detectors as the number of slices, and some yield as many slices with fewer numbers of detectors (uniquely switching x-ray beams on the fly). In either case, in the past decade (1998–2008) we have witnessed rapid technological developments with evolutionary leaps in the MDCT applications.

According to surveys, nearly 80% of all CT scans performed are routine head, chest, abdomen, and pelvis (HCAP) scans, for which the current MDCT systems have more than sufficient spatial and temporal resolution. Faster scanning and improved spatial resolution have benefited newer clinical applications, including vascular imaging applications. The main beneficiary of 64-slice MDCT scanners has been cardiac imaging. The greater spatial and temporal resolution has greatly improved the quality of coronary CT studies. Many studies and policies developed by health insurance reimbursement groups favor and in some instances recommend (few go as far as mandating) the use of 64-slice MDCT scanners for cardiac applications. Yet, the ability to scan an entire organ (the heart) in a single rotation and still maintaining high spatial and temporal resolution is further fueling the development of MDCT scanners. Now that the target of capturing an organ (heart) with a single scan is met to some extent, the future is more challenging and exciting and difficult to forecast. However, future trends in MDCT can be found in the following areas detailed in this chapter.

Dual-Energy Applications

The introduction of the dual-source CT scanner (DSCT) peaked the interest in energy-dependent imaging. The concept of dual-energy imaging to delineate differences in x-ray absorption characteristics has been in existence for a long time, even from the time of early generation of CT scanners. The dual-energy CT (DECT) technique involves separating the information gained on imaging from x-ray photons of different energies. Characteristic attenuation profiles are then used to separate materials such as bone, soft tissue, and contrast media. This paves way to transform an imaging modality that provides anatomical-only information to an imaging modality that provides both anatomical and functional types of information.

Dual-source CT scanners have made dual-energy CT scanning easier and more clinically feasible. With DSCT scanners, it is easier to

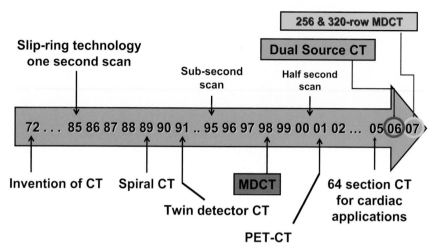

Figure 12.1. Timeline showing the various developmental milestones in the field of CT.

perform dual-energy scans, with each x-ray tube set to a different tube voltage. At the same time, several other CT manufacturers have developed DECT applications with the existing MDCT scanners (single x-ray tube), either by switching-tube voltages (kVp) at every point along with fast response detectors or by constant-tube voltage with two detectors placed on top of each other with energy discriminating capability or by using photon counting detector technology. Many new clinical applications are in development, with a few are in the validation process, and all signs are indicating that DECT application, although is in its infancy, carries great potential for long-term growth.

Radiation Dose

Radiation dose from CT procedures are of concern, especially with the rapid growth in the number of CT scanners both in the United States and worldwide. According to National Council of Radiation Protection Scientific Committee 6-2 study*, in 2006, the effective dose to the U.S. population from medical radiation exposure has increased by nearly 600% in the past 25 years. Examining further the increase in overall effective dose to the U.S. population, it is not surprising to find that the effective dose from CT procedures dominates by nearly 50% the contribution from all medical radiation exposure (Fig. 12.2). Although this information

has no minimal bearing on the individual risks for patients undergoing CT procedures, it draws attention to the overall radiation burden to the population from CT procedures.

The advances in MDCT technology have led to many new clinical applications, along with the proliferation of MDCT scanners. In fact, according to a survey in 2007, there are more than 10,000 CT scanners in the United States alone and, among them, 80% are MDCT scanners. Similar trends in the overall increase in number of CT procedures and number of MDCT scanners worldwide are evident. This increase in overall CT procedures and number of scanners draw and will continue to draw special attention to the issue of radiation dose. The information about the effective dose from CT and other x-ray imaging modalities is useful for examining epidemiological risk to the population; however, it does not apply unilaterally to the individual patients getting CT scans. At the individual level, it is important to understand the benefits and the accompanying risks as applied to a particular instance. As long as the benefits from a CT procedure outweigh the risks, performing CT scanning is always advantageous in terms of diagnosis and proper treatment. The difficulty is assessing benefits and risks for each CT scanning and it is a daunting task, especially when there are so many repeat CT scans. Repeat CT scans are getting more attention and in fact warrant special scrutiny.

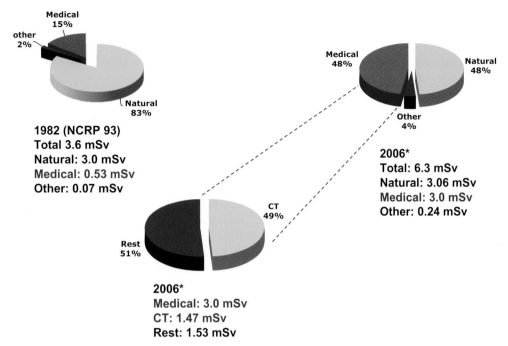

Figure 12.2. Effective dose per person for the U.S. population in 2006*. The contribution from CT is 49% of all the medical radiation exposure.
*Mettler FA, et al., Health Physics. 2008;95:502–507.

The establishment of the appropriateness of a CT scan based on benefits and risks will be one of key areas of development in the near future.

Efforts to lower radiation dose with MDCT protocols by optimizing scan techniques in various protocols will become one of the priorities among the future trends in MDCT in the near future. Along with this, further refinement in dose-modulation strategies will be key. For a long time, radiation dose was not on the radar among users (clinicians) and providers (manufacturers). However, with recent media attention and as the subject of many studies, the radiation dose issue is in the limelight and is now considered a key component of the technology, drawing special attention from all players, including users (clinicians), providers (manufacturers) and even regulators (gatekeepers).

Another area that is drawing special attention is the methodology used in measuring CT dose. Even though CT dose measurements have always been performed with 16 cm and 32 cm circular phantoms using 100-mm pencil chambers, the arrival of 256- and 320-row MDCT scanners with an x-ray beam width of 14–16 cm in longitudinal direction has introduced greater challenges for the medical physics community to develop standards for dose measurements and the evaluation of image quality.

Also of importance are the efforts to reduce radiation dose that are leading to the development of new types of image reconstruction algorithms. One such method is *iterative reconstruction*, which is used commonly in nuclear medicine imaging procedures and was thought not to be feasible for CT image reconstruction because of slow computing time. However, with attention drawn toward radiation dose from MDCT protocols in addition to the development of faster computer processors, many efforts are underway to develop image reconstruction algorithms with iterative reconstruction principles. With iterative reconstruction methods, it has been shown that it is possible to reduce radiation dose for protocols without compromise in image quality. Second, with increasing demand for greater number of slices per gantry rotation, the x-ray beam width is increasing, resulting in increased cone beam angle. This increase in cone beam angle creates unacceptable cone beam artifacts in existing image reconstruction algorithms and therefore the increasing cone beam demands a new type of reconstruction algorithm.

Whole-Body CT Screening

MDCT technology has made whole-body CT screening feasible and, in fact, whole-body CT screening for asymptomatic subjects has generated many controversies. Whole-body CT screening of asymptomatic subjects have raised concern as a result of the absence of well-documented benefits that outweigh the radiation risk associated with such scans. In addition, whole-body CT screening at low doses has shown to result in more false-positive results in subjects, resulting in additional CT scans that often find true negatives but expose subjects to additional doses of radiation. In fact, the position statements from various professional societies against the whole-body CT screening of asymptomatic subjects and excessive competition among the centers providing such scans in addition to global and local economic conditions have impacted and resulted in overall reduction in such scans. However, if the benefits from such scans can be demonstrated with proper clinical trials, then whole-body CT screening may be recommended for routine evaluation for asymptomatic subjects.

Only recently, virtual colonoscopy procedures that are possible with MDCT technology have been shown to be as effective in regular colonoscopy procedures. Despite the radiation risk associated with virtual colonoscopy, it is now considered as an alternative to regular colonoscopy procedures and is recommended for annual screening for elderly subjects (Every 5 years starting at age 50 y. 2009 American Cancer Society, Recommendations. CA Cancer J Clin 2009;59:27–41). Similar studies to establish the benefits of whole-body CT screening are required and may be in the works. In time and once the benefits are established, the whole-body CT scanning may become a "one-stop" evaluation center and may have the potential to reduce additional scans and impact in lowering overall radiation burden and may help in lowering the ever-bulging health care costs.

Flat-Panel CT

With the goal of capturing an entire organ system, efforts are underway to develop flat-panel CT. In fact, prototypes of flat-panel CT scanners with flat-panel detectors of 30 cm by 45 cm are in developmental stage, but there are many challenges that are to be overcome before such scanners become clinically feasible. Among them are increased scatter radiation caused by large field size, impacting low-contrast resolution (hallmark advantage of CT). The increase in scatter radiation demands the introduction of some type of grid to cleanup the scatter, which in turn will demand an increase in radiation dose. Also, the demand for greater spatial resolution with smaller pixel size with flat panel requires increasing the radiation dose. Because the radiation dose in CT is already drawing much attention, it is an uphill battle to introduce such flat-panel CT scanners to clinical use unless the aforementioned challenges are resolved.

Meanwhile, variations of flat-panel CT designs have resulted in obtaining CT-type images with the use of regular radiographic and fluoroscopic systems. For example, interventional fluoroscopy systems with flat-panel devices are now capable of producing CT-like images. Modern interventional fluoroscopy systems with flat-panel image receptors are capable of acquiring images during rotational angiography procedures and, with special reconstruction algorithms, yield CT-like images. However, the scan time is longer, that is, on the order of few seconds compared with less than half-a-second with MDCT scanners. The temporal resolution and spatial resolution is much lower than that obtained with MDCT scanners, and the radiation dose can be quite high. However, the unique advantage of CT-like imaging with an interventional fluoroscopy system is that the patient undergoing interventional procedure can now be evaluated immediately after the interventional procedure and doesn't have to be relocated to a CT scanner.

Niche Markets for CT with Special Applications

Cone-beam CT yielding CT-like imaging is gaining more acceptance in radiation oncology departments. Cone-beam CT scanning often includes an x-ray tube and a flat-panel device that are positioned orthogonal to the radiation treatment systems such as linear accelerator. Cone beam CT imaging is performed to verify the location of radiation treatment and is proving very beneficial for image-guided radiation therapy.

Similarly, cone-beam CT technology is finding rapid growth potential in special areas such as dentistry and neurology. Cone-beam CT is well suited for imaging the craniofacial area and, with inexpensive x-ray tubes, high-quality detector systems and powerful personal computers, such systems are becoming more affordable and commercially available. Already there are several cone-beam CT scanners commercially available that are finding or creating niche markets such as dental CT and neuro-CT scanners.

Small-animal imaging is another area in which micro-CT scanners are used in hybrid imaging systems along with positron emission tomography or single-photon emission computed tomography systems. Micro-CT scanners use low-power x-ray tubes with flat-panel devices and provide anatomical locations, whereas positron emission tomography or single-photon emission computed tomography systems are used to obtain functional information. With the growing importance of molecular imaging, further developments in small-animal imaging systems can be expected in the future.

Conclusions

In the four decades since CT became available, there were times when it was a popular notion that "CT is dead." However, each time before the notion became a reality, the technological advances propelled the field of CT imaging much stronger and robust. First, the introduction helical CT that led to continuous acquisition in the 1980s and next the introduction of MDCT in later 1990s have dismantled such illusions. In fact, the field of CT appears to be still in its infancy and has so much more room for development. The current development in both hardware and software is transforming the field of CT from being the provider of only anatomical information to becoming a provider of both anatomical and functional imaging systems. With current MDCT scanners capable of generating larger number of slices at a fast rate and with growing concerns for radiation dose with MDCT, it appears we may be seeing the end of slice wars and witnessing the beginning of dose wars. In fact it is beneficial for the field of CT imaging if dose wars gain more strength and result in imaging procedures that can be considered as low-dose procedures in future. The ballpark analogy of "you build, they will come" also has been true in CT, especially with MDCT technology. With MDCT technology, many a times it appears as if "the solution (MDCT scanner) is searching for a problem (clinical application)." With the technology capable of performing faster and finer imaging, many new clinical applications are developed and many more are been developed.

Personally, I have experienced the rollercoaster ride of CT technology these past few years and expect similar excitement in the field of CT for years to come. CT is alive and well and has widely changed the landscape of diagnosis and continues to change the field of diagnosis and treatment for years to come.

APPENDIX

I

Suggested Readings

1. AAPM (American Association of Physicists in Medicine), Specification and Acceptance Testing of Computed Tomography Scanners. Task Group Report 2. College Park, MD: American Association of Physicists in Medicine, 1993. Available at: http://www.aapm.org/pubs/reports/RPT_39.pdf. Accessed February 18, 2009.

2. AAPM (American Association of Physicists in Medicine), The Measurement, Reporting and Management of Radiation Dose in CT, Task Group Report 96. College Park, MD: Association of Physicists in Medicine; 2003. Available at: http://www.aapm.org/pubs/reports/RPT_96.pdf. Accessed February 18, 2009.

3. NAS/NRC (National Academy of Sciences/National Research Council), Health Risks From Exposure to Low Levels of Ionizing Radiation, BEIR V. Washington, DC: National Academy Press; 1990.

4. ICRP 1991 Recommendations of the International Commission on Radiological Protection. ICRP publication 60. Ann ICRP 1991; 21(1–3).

5. NAS/NRC (National Academy of Sciences/National Research Council), Health Risks From Exposure to Low Levels of Ionizing Radiation, BEIR VII, Phase 2. Washington, DC: National Academy Press; 2006.

6. NCRP (National Council on Radiation Protection and Measurements), Ionizing Radiation Exposure of the Population of the United States, NCRP Report No. 93. Bethesda, MD: National Council on Radiation Protection and Measurements; 1987.

7. NCRP (National Council of Radiation Protection and Measurements), Limitation of Exposure to Ionizing Radiation, NCRP Report No. 116. Bethesda, MD: National Council of Radiation Protection and Measurements; 1993.

8. NCRP (National Council on Radiation Protection and Measurements), Structural Shielding Design for Medical X-ray Imaging Facilities. NCRP Report No. 147. Bethesda, MD: National Council on Radiation Protection and Measurements, Bethesda; 2004.

9. The 2007 Recommendations of the International Commission on Radiological Protection. ICRP publication 103. Ann ICRP 2007; 37:1–332.

10. Amis ES Jr., Butler PF, Applegate KE, et al. American College of Radiology white paper on radiation dose in medicine. *J Am Coll Radiol.* 2007; 4:272–284.

11. Ammann E, Kutschera W. X-ray tubes—continuous innovative technology. *Br J Radiol.* 1997; 70 Spec No:S1–S9.

12. Baum U, Anders K, Steinbichler G, et al. Improvement of image quality of multislice spiral CT scans of the head and neck region using a raw database-based multidimensional adaptive filtering (MAF) technique. *Eur Radiol.* 2004;14:1873–1881.

13. Becker CR, Jakobs TF, Aydemir S, et al. Helical and single-slice conventional CT versus electron beam CT for the quantification of coronary artery calcification. *AJR Am J Roentgenol.* 2000; 174:543–547.

14. Becker CR, Kleffel T, Crispin A, et al. Coronary artery calcium measurement: agreement of multirow detector and electron beam CT. *AJR Am J Roentgenol.* 2001; 176:1295–1298.

15. Becker CR, Knez A, Leber A, et al. Detection of coronary artery stenoses with multislice helical CT angiography. *J Comput Assist Tomogr.* 2002; 26:750–755.

16. Bild DE, Detrano R, Peterson D, et al. Ethnic differences in coronary calcification: the Multi-Ethnic Study of Atherosclerosis (MESA). *Circulation.* 2005; 111:1313–20.

17. Blodgett TM, Meltzer CC, Townsend DW. PET/CT: form and function. *Radiology*. 2007; 242:360–385.

18. Boiselle PM, Hasegawa I, Nishino M, et al. Comparison of artifacts on coronal reformation and axial CT pulmonary angiography images using single-detector and 4- and 8-detector multidetector-row helical CT scanners. *Acad Radiol*. 2005; 12:602–607.

19. Bomma C, Dalal D, Tandri H, et al. Evolving role of multidetector computed tomography in evaluation of arrhythmogenic right ventricular dysplasia/cardiomyopathy. *Am J Cardiol*. 2007; 100:99–105.

20. Brenner D, Elliston C, Hall E, Berdon W. Estimated risks of radiation-induced fatal cancer from pediatric CT. *AJR Am J Roentgenol*. 2001; 176:289–296.

21. Brenner DJ. Radiation risks potentially associated with low-dose CT screening of adult smokers for lung cancer. *Radiology*. 2004; 231:440–445.

22. Brenner DJ. Is it time to retire the CTDI for CT quality assurance and dose optimization? [Letter] *Med Phys* 2005; 32:3225–3226.

23. Brenner DJ, Elliston CD. Estimated radiation risks potentially associated with full-body CT screening. *Radiology*. 2004; 232:735–738.

24. Brenner DJ, Hall EJ. Computed tomography—an increasing source of radiation exposure. *N Engl J Med*. 2007; 357:2277–2284.

25. Brenner DJ, Mossman KL. Do radiation doses below 1 cGy increase cancer risks? *Radiat Res*. 2005; 163:692–693.

26. Brisse HJ, Madec L, Gaboriaud G, et al. Automatic exposure control in multichannel CT with tube current modulation to achieve a constant level of image noise: experimental assessment on pediatric phantoms. *Med Phys*. 2007; 34:3018–3033.

27. Brix G, Nagel HD, Stamm G, et al. Radiation exposure in multi-slice versus single-slice spiral CT: results of a nationwide survey. *Eur Radiol*. 2003; 13:1979–1991.

28. Brix G, Nissen-Meyer S, Lechel U, et al. Radiation exposures of cancer patients from medical X-rays: How relevant are they for individual patients and population exposure? *Eur J Radiol*., 2008 August 21.

29. Budoff MJ, Achenbach S, Duerinckx A. Clinical utility of computed tomography and magnetic resonance techniques for noninvasive coronary angiography. *J Am Coll Cardiol*. 2003; 42:1867–1878.

30. Bushberg JT, Siebert JA, Leidholdt EM, et al. *The Essential Physics of Medical Imaging*. Baltimore: Lippincott Williams and Wilkins; 2002.

31. Choi HS, Choi BW, Choe KO, et al. Pitfalls, artifacts, and remedies in multi- detector row CT coronary angiography. *Radiographics*. 2004; 24:787–800.

32. Cody DD, Mahesh M. AAPM/RSNA physics tutorial for residents: technologic advances in multidetector CT with a focus on cardiac imaging. *Radiographics*. 2007; 27:1829–1837.

33. Cody DD, Moxley DM, Krugh KT, et al. Strategies for formulating appropriate MDCT techniques when imaging the chest, abdomen, and pelvis in pediatric patients. *AJR Am J Roentgenol*. 2004; 182:849–859.

34. Cohade C, Osman M, Nakamoto Y, et al. Initial experience with oral contrast in PET/CT: phantom and clinical studies. *J Nucl Med*. 2003; 44:412–416.

35. Cohade C, Wahl RL. Applications of positron emission tomography/computed tomography image fusion in clinical positron emission tomography-clinical use, interpretation methods, diagnostic improvements. *Semin Nucl Med*. 2003; 33:228–237.

36. Crawford CR, King KF. Computed tomography scanning with simultaneous patient translation. *Med Phys*. 1990; 17:967–982.

37. de Denaro M, Bregant P, Severgnini M, de Guarrini F. In vivo dosimetry for estimation of effective doses in multislice CT coronary angiography. *Med Phys*. 2007; 34:3705–3710.

38. Deak P, van Straten M, Shrimpton PC, Zankl M, Kalender WA. Validation of a Monte Carlo tool for patient-specific dose simulations in multi-slice computed tomography. *Eur Radiol*. 2008; 18:759–772.

39. Desjardins B, Kazerooni EA. ECG-gated cardiac CT. *AJR Am J Roentgenol*. 2004; 182:993–1010.

40. Detrano RC. Coronary artery scanning using electron beam computed tomography. *Am J Card Imaging*. 1996; 10:97–100.

41. Dixon RL. A new look at CT dose measurement: beyond CTDI. *Med Phys*. 2003; 30:1272–1280.

42. Dixon RL. Restructuring CT dosimetry—a realistic strategy for the future Requiem for the pencil chamber. *Med Phys*. 2006; 33:3973–3976.

43. Earls JP, Berman EL, Urban BA, et al. Prospectively gated transverse coronary CT angiography versus retrospectively gated helical technique: improved image quality and reduced radiation dose. *Radiology*. 2008; 246:742–753.

44. Einstein AJ, Henzlova MJ, Rajagopalan S. Estimating risk of cancer associated with radiation exposure from 64-slice computed tomography coronary angiography. *Jama.* 2007; 298:317–323.

45. Fayad ZA, Fuster V, Nikolaou K, Becker C. Computed tomography and magnetic resonance imaging for noninvasive coronary angiography and plaque imaging: current and potential future concepts. *Circulation.* 2002; 106:2026–2034.

46. Felmlee JP, Gray JE, Leetzow ML, Price JC. Estimated fetal radiation dose from multislice CT studies. *AJR Am J Roentgenol.* 1990; 154:185–190.

47. Fishman EK, Kuszyk B. 3D imaging: musculoskeletal applications. *Crit Rev Diagn Imaging.* 2001; 42:59–100.

48. Fishman EK, Magid D, Ney DR, et al. Three-dimensional imaging. *Radiology.* 1991; 181: 321–337.

49. Johnson PT, Fishman EK. IV Contrast selection for MDCT: current thoughts and practice. *AJR Am J Roentgenol.* 2006:406–415.

50. Flohr T, Stierstorfer K, Bruder H, et al. Image reconstruction and image quality evaluation for a 16-slice CT scanner. *Med Phys.* 2003; 30:832–845.

51. Flohr T, Stierstorfer K, Raupach R, et al. Performance evaluation of a 64-slice CT system with z-flying focal spot. *Rofo.* 2004; 176:1803–1810.

52. Flohr TG, Joseph Schoepf U, Ohnesorge BM. Chasing the heart: new developments for cardiac CT. *J Thorac Imaging.* 2007; 22:4–16.

53. Flohr TG, McCollough CH, Bruder H, et al. First performance evaluation of a dual-source CT (DSCT) system. *Eur Radiol.* 2006; 16:256–268.

54. Flohr TG, Schaller S, Stierstorfer K, et al. Multi-detector row CT systems and image-reconstruction techniques. *Radiology.* 2005; 235:756–773.

55. Flohr TG, Stierstorfer K, Suss C, et al. Novel ultrahigh resolution data acquisition and image reconstruction for multi-detector row CT. *Med Phys.* 2007; 34:1712–1723.

56. Flohr TG, Stierstorfer K, Ulzheimer S, et al. Image reconstruction and image quality evaluation for a 64-slice CT scanner with z-flying focal spot. *Med Phys.* 2005; 32:2536–2547.

57. Fox SH, ed. *CT Tube Technology.* Madison: Advanced Medical Publishing, 1995.

58. Frush D. Strategies of dose reduction. *Pediatr Radiol.* 2002; 32:293–297.

59. Frush D. CT and radiation risks: what pediatric health care providers should know. *Pediatrics.* 2003; 112:289–291.

60. Frush D. Computed tomography: important considerations for pediatric patients. *Expert Rev Med Devices.* 2005; 2:567–575.

61. Gerber B, Rosen BD, Mahesh M, et al. Physical Principles of Cardiovascular Imaging. In: St. John Sutton M, Rutherford J, eds. *Clinical Cardiovascular Imaging: A Companion to Braunwald's Heart Disease.* Philadelphia: Elsevier-Saunders; 2004:1–77.

62. Gerber TC, Kuzo RS, Morin RL. Techniques and parameters for estimating radiation exposure and dose in cardiac computed tomography. *Int J Cardiovasc Imaging.* 2005; 21:165–176.

63. Gerber TC, Stratmann BP, Kuzo RS, et al. Effect of acquisition technique on radiation dose and image quality in multidetector row computed tomography coronary angiography with submillimeter collimation. *Invest Radiol.* 2005; 40:556–563.

64. Gies M, Kalender WA, Wolf H, et al. Dose reduction in CT by anatomically adapted tube current modulation. I. Simulation studies. *Med Phys.* 1999; 26:2235–2247.

65. Goske MJ, Applegate KE, Boylan J, et al. Image Gently(SM): a national education and communication campaign in radiology using the science of social marketing. *J Am Coll Radiol.* 2008; 5:1200–1205.

66. Gralla J, Spycher F, Pignolet C, et al. Evaluation of a 16-MDCT scanner in an emergency department: initial clinical experience and workflow analysis. *AJR Am J Roentgenol.* 2005; 185:232–238.

67. Grass M, Manzke R, Nielsen T, et al. Helical cardiac cone beam reconstruction using retrospective ECG gating. *Phys Med Biol.* 2003; 48: 3069–3084.

68. Hall EJ, Brenner DJ. Cancer risks from diagnostic radiology. *Br J Radiol.* 2008; 81:362–378.

69. Husmann L, Valenta I, Gaemperli O, et al. Feasibility of low-dose coronary CT angiography: first experience with prospective ECG-gating, *Euro Heart J,* 2008; 29:191–197.

70. Hendee WR, Ritenour R. *Medical Imaging Physics.* St. Louis: Mosby; 1992.

71. Herzog C, Mulvihill DM, Nguyen SA, et al. Pediatric cardiovascular CT angiography: radiation dose reduction using automatic anatomic tube current modulation. *AJR Am J Roentgenol.* 2008; 190:1232–1240.

72. Heuschmid M, Kuettner A, Schroeder S, et al. ECG-gated 16-MDCT of the coronary arteries: assessment of image quality and accuracy in detecting stenoses. *AJR Am J Roentgenol.* 2005; 184:1413–1419.

73. Hofer M. *CT Teaching—A Systematic Approach to CT Reading.* Stuttgart, Germany: Thieme; 2003.

74. Hoffmann MH, Shi H, Schmid FT, et al. Noninvasive coronary imaging with MDCT in comparison to invasive conventional coronary angiography: a fast-developing technology. *AJR Am J Roentgenol.* 2004; 182:601–608.

75. Hohl C, Suess C, Wildberger JE, et al. Dose reduction during CT fluoroscopy: phantom study of angular beam modulation. *Radiology.* 2008; 246:519–525.

76. Hounsfield GN. Historical notes on computerized axial tomography. *J Can Assoc Radiol.* 1976; 27:135–142.

77. Hounsfield GN. Nobel Award address. Computed medical imaging. *Med Phys.* 1980; 7:283–290.

78. Hounsfield GN. Computerized transverse axial scanning (tomography): Part I. Description of system. 1973. *Br J Radiol.* 1995; 68:H166–H172.

79. Hsieh J. A general approach to the reconstruction of x-ray helical computed tomography. *Med Phys.* 1996; 23:221–229.

80. Hsieh J. Analytical models for multi-slice helical CT performance parameters. *Med Phys.* 2003; 30:169–178.

81. Hsieh J. *Computed Tomography—Principles, Design, Artifacts and Recent Advances.* Bellingham, WA: SPIE-The International Society for Optical Engineering; 2003.

82. Hsieh J, Londt J, Vass M, et al. Step-and-shoot data acquisition and reconstruction for cardiac x-ray computed tomography. *Med Phys.* 2006; 33:4236–4248.

83. Hu H. Multi-slice helical CT: scan and reconstruction. *Med Phys.* 1999; 26:5–18.

84. Huda W, Vance A. Patient radiation doses from adult and pediatric CT. *AJR Am J Roentgenol.* 2007; 188:540–546.

85. Hui H, Pan T, Shen Y. Multislice helical CT: image temporal resolution. *IEEE Trans Med Imaging.* 2000; 19:384–390.

86. Hundt W, Siebert K, Wintersperger BJ, et al. Assessment of global left ventricular function: comparison of cardiac multidetector-row computed tomography with angiocardiography. *J Comput Assist Tomogr.* 2005; 29:373–381.

87. Hunold P, Vogt FM, Schmermund A, et al. Radiation exposure during cardiac CT: effective doses at multi-detector row CT and electron-beam CT. *Radiology.* 2003; 226:145–152.

88. IEC. Medical Electrical Equipment. part 2-44: Particular Requirements for the Safety of X-ray Equipment for Computed Tomography.

Geneva, Switzerland: IEC Publications No. 60601–2-44; 2002.

89. ImPACT Technology Update. Multi-Slice CT Scanners. London: ImPACT; 1999.

90. Jakobs TF, Becker CR, Ohnesorge B, et al. Multi-slice helical CT of the heart with retrospective ECG gating: reduction of radiation exposure by ECG-controlled tube current modulation. *Eur Radiol.* 2002; 12:1081–1086.

91. Javadi M, Mahesh M, McBride G, et al. Lowering radiation dose for integrated assessment of coronary morphology and physiology: first experience with step-and-shoot CT angiography in a rubidium 82 PET-CT protocol. *J Nucl Cardiol.* 2008; 15:783–790.

92. Jennifer C. O'Daniel DMS, Dianna D. Cody. Reducing radiation exposure from survey CT scans. *AJR Am J Roentgenol.* 2005:509–515.

93. John M. Boone EMG, J. Anthony Seibert, Sandra L. Wootton-Gorges. Dose reduction in pediatric CT: a rational approach. *Radiology.* 2003; 228:352.

94. Johnson PT, Horton KM, Mahesh M, Fishman EK. Multidetector computed tomography for suspected appendicitis: multi-institutional survey of 16-MDCT data acquisition protocols and review of pertinent literature. *J Comput Assist Tomogr.* 2006; 30:758–764.

95. Justin Campbell MKK, Rizzo S, Maher MM, Shepard J. Scanning beyond anatomic limits of the thorax in chest CT: Findings, radiation dose, and automatic tube current modulation. *AJR Am J Roentgenol.* 2005:1525–1530.

96. Kacherliess M, Schaller S, and Kalender W. Advanced single slice rebinning in cone beam spiral CT. *Med Phys.* 2000; 27: 754–772.

97. Kachelriess M, Ulzheimer S, Kalender WA. ECG-correlated image reconstruction from sub-second multi-slice spiral CT scans of the heart. *Med Phys.* 2000; 27:1881–1902.

98. Kalender WA. Thin-section three-dimensional spiral CT: is isotropic imaging possible? *Radiology.* 1995; 197:578–580.

99. Kalender WA. *Computed Tomography—Fundamentals, System Technology, Image Quality, Applications.* Erlangen, Germany: Publicis Corporate Publishing; 2005.

100. Kalender WA, Buchenau S, Deak P, et al. Technical approaches to the optimisation of CT. *Phys Med.* 2008; 24:71–79.

101. Kalender WA, Polacin A. Physical performance characteristics of spiral CT scanning. *Med Phys.* 1991; 18:910–915.

102. Kalender WA, Schmidt B, Zankl M, et al. A PC program for estimating organ dose and effective

dose values in computed tomography. *Eur Radiol.* 1999; 9:555–562.

103. Kalender WA, Seissler W, Klotz E, et al. Spiral volumetric CT with single-breath-hold technique, continuous transport, and continuous scanner rotation. *Radiology.* 1990; 176:181–183.

104. Kalender WA, Wolf H, Suess C. Dose reduction in CT by anatomically adapted tube current modulation. II. Phantom measurements. *Med Phys.* 1999; 26:2248–2253.

105. Kalra M, Maher MM, Toth TL, et al. Radiation from "extra" images acquired with abdominal and/or pelvic CT: effect of automatic tube current modulation. *Radiology.* 2004; 232:409–414.

106. Kalra M, Maher MM, Toth TL, Leena et al. Strategies for CT radiation dose optimization. *Radiology.* 2004; 230:619–628.

107. Kalra MK, Maher MM, Toth TL, et al. Techniques and applications of automatic tube current modulation for CT. *Radiology.* 2004; 233:649–657.

108. Katsevich A. Analysis of an exact inversion algorithm for spiral cone beam CT. *Phys Med Biol.* 2002; 47: 2583–2598.

109. Khursheed A, Hillier MC, Shrimpton PC, et al. Influence of patient age on normalized effective doses calculated for CT examinations. *Br J Radiol.* 2002; 75:819–830.

110. Kinahan PE, Townsend DW, Beyer T, et al. Attenuation correction for a combined 3D PET/CT scanner. *Med Phys.* 1998; 25:2046–2053.

111. Klingenbeck-Regn K, Flohr T, Ohnesorge B, et al. Strategies for cardiac CT imaging. *Int J Cardiovasc Imaging.* 2002; 18:143–151.

112. Klingenbeck-Regn K, Schaller S, Flohr T, et al. Subsecond multi-slice computed tomography: basics and applications. Eur *J Radiol.* 1999; 31:110–124.

113. Knollmen F, Coakley F. *Multislice CT.* Philadelphia: Saunders-Elsevier; 2006.

114. Lee CI, Haims AH, Monico EP, et al. Diagnostic CT scans: assessment of patient, physician, and radiologist awareness of radiation dose and possible risks. *Radiology.* 2004; 231:393–398.

115. Linton OW, Mettler FA Jr. National conference on dose reduction in CT, with an emphasis on pediatric patients. *AJR Am J Roentgenol.* 2003; 181:321–329.

116. Ludlow JB, Ivanovic M. Comparative dosimetry of dental CBCT devices and 64-slice CT for oral and maxillofacial radiology. *Oral Surg Oral Med Oral Pathol Oral Radiol Endod.* 2008; 106:106–114.

117. Mahesh M. Search for isotropic resolution in CT from conventional through multiple-row detector. *Radiographics.* 2002; 22:949–962.

118. Mahesh M. Next-generation x-ray CT units will provide <500 msec images with 3D resolution comparable to today's projection radiography. For the proposition. *Med Phys.* 2003; 30: 1543–1544.

119. Mahesh M. Cardiac Imaging—technical advances in MDCT compared with conventional X-ray angiography. In: Boulton E, ed. US Cardiology 2006. *The Authoritative Review of the Clinical and Scientific Issues Relating to Cardiology With Perspectives on the Future.* London, UK: Touch Briefings (www.touchcardiology.com); 2006:115–119.

120. Mahesh M. Slice Wars versus Dose Wars in Multiple-row Detector CT. *J Am Coll Radiol.* 2009; In Press.

121. Mahesh M, Cody DD. Physics of cardiac imaging with multiple-row detector CT. *Radiographics.* 2007; 27:1495–1509.

122. Mahesh M, Scatarige JC, Cooper J, Fishman EK. Dose and pitch relationship for a particular multislice CT scanner. *AJR Am J Roentgenol.* 2001; 177:1273–1275.

123. Mahnken AH, Wildberger JE, Koos R, Gunther RW. Multislice spiral computed tomography of the heart: technique, current applications, and perspective. *Cardiovasc Intervent Radiol.* 2005; 28:388–399.

124. Martin CJ. Effective dose: how should it be applied to medical exposures? *Br J Radiol.* 2007; 80:639–647.

125. McCollough CH. Patient dose in cardiac computed tomography. *Herz.* 2003; 28:1–6.

126. McCollough CH, Bruesewitz MR, McNitt-Gray MF, et al. The phantom portion of the American College of Radiology (ACR) computed tomography (CT) accreditation program: practical tips, artifact examples, and pitfalls to avoid. *Med Phys.* 2004; 31:2423–2442.

127. McCollough CH, Schueler BA. Calculation of effective dose. *Med Phys.* 2000; 27:828–837.

128. McCollough CH, Zink FE. Performance evaluation of a multi-slice CT system. *Med Phys.* 1999; 26:2223–2230.

129. McLean D, Malitz N, Lewis S. Survey of effective dose levels from typical paediatric CT protocols. *Australas Radiol.* 2003; 47:135–142.

130. McNitt-Gray MF, Cagnon CH, Solberg TD, et al. Radiation dose in Spiral CT: The relative effects of collimation and pitch. *Med Phys.* 1999; 26:409–414.

131. Menke J. Comparison of different body size parameters for individual dose adaptation in body CT of adults. *Radiology.* 2005; 236:565–571.

132. Mettler FA Jr., Huda W, Yoshizumi TT, et al. Effective doses in radiology and diagnostic nuclear medicine: a catalog. *Radiology.* 2008; 248:254–263.

133. Mettler FA Jr., Thomadsen BR, Bhargavan M, et al. Medical radiation exposure in the U.S. in 2006: preliminary results. *Health Phys.* 2008; 95:502–507.

134. Michael G, Kalender WA, Wolf H, and Suess C. Dose Reduction in CT Anatomically Adapted Tube Current Modulation. *Med Phys.* 1999; 26: 2235–2247.

135. Morgan HT. Dose reduction for CT pediatric imaging. *Pediat Radiol.* 2002; 32:724–728.

136. Morgan-Hughes GJ, Marshall AJ, Roobottom CA. Multislice computed tomography cardiac imaging: current status. *Clin Radiol.* 2002; 57:872–882.

137. Mori S, Endo M, Obata T, et al. Clinical potentials of the prototype 256-detector row CT-scanner. *Acad Radiol.* 2005; 12:148–154.

138. Morin RL, Gerber TC, McCollough CH. Radiation dose in computed tomography of the heart. *Circulation.* 2003; 107:917–922.

139. Nagel HD, ed. *Radiation Exposure in Computed Tomography: Fundamentals, Influencing Parameters, Dose Assessment, Optimisation, Scanner Data, Terminology.* Hamburg: COCIR; 2002.

140. Nakanishi T, Kayashima Y, Inoue R, et al. Pitfalls in 16-detector row CT of the coronary arteries. *Radiographics.* 2005; 25:425–438; discussion 438–440.

141. Nasir K, Budoff MJ, Post WS, et al. Electron beam CT versus helical CT scans for assessing coronary calcification: current utility and future directions. *Am Heart J.* 2003; 146:969–977.

142. Nickoloff E, Dutta AK, Lu ZF. Influence of phantom diameter, kVp and scan mode upon computed tomography dose index. *Med Phys.* 2003; 30:395.

143. Nickoloff EL, Alderson PO. Radiation exposures to patients from CT: reality, public perception, and policy. *AJR Am J Roentgenol.* 2001; 177: 285–287.

144. Nieman K, van Ooijen P, Rensing B, et al. Four-dimensional cardiac imaging with multislice computed tomography. *Circulation.* 2001; 103:E62.

145. Nikolaou K, Flohr T, Knez A, et al. Advances in cardiac CT imaging: 64-slice scanner. Int *J Cardiovasc Imaging.* 2004; 20:535–540.

146. Nikolaou K, Flohr T, Stierstorfer K, et al. Flat panel computed tomography of human ex vivo heart and bone specimens: initial experience. *Eur Radiol.* 2005; 15:329–333.

147. Ohnesorge B, Flohr T, Fischbach R, et al. Reproducibility of coronary calcium quantification in repeat examinations with retrospectively ECG-gated multisection spiral CT. *Eur Radiol.* 2002; 12:1532–1540.

148. Ohnesorge BM, Hofmann LK, Flohr TG, et al. CT for imaging coronary artery disease: defining the paradigm for its application. *Int J Cardiovasc Imaging* 2005; 21:85–104.

149. Osman MM, Cohade C, Nakamoto Y, et al. Respiratory motion artifacts on PET emission images obtained using CT attenuation correction on PET-CT. *Eur J Nucl Med Mol. Imaging* 2003; 30:603–606.

150. Pages J, Buls N, Osteaux M. CT doses in children: a multicentre study. *Br J Radiol.* 2003; 76:803–811.

151. Pandharipande P, Krinsky, GA, Rusinek, H, et al. Perfusion imaging of the liver: current challenges and future goals. *Radiology.* 2005; 234:661–673.

152. Pannu HK, Alvarez W Jr., Fishman EK. Beta-blockers for cardiac CT: a primer for the radiologist. *AJR Am J Roentgenol.* 2006; 186:S341–345.

153. Pannu HK, Flohr TG, Corl FM, et al. Current concepts in multi-detector row CT evaluation of the coronary arteries: principles, techniques, and anatomy. *Radiographics* 2003; 23 Spec No:S111–125.

154. Pannu HK, Jacobs JE, Lai S, et al. Coronary CT angiography with 64-MDCT: assessment of vessel visibility. *AJR Am J Roentgenol.* 2006; 187:119–126.

155. Philips Medical Systems. Philips DoseWise: What's behind the perfect image? Andover, MA: Philips Healthcare, US; 2004.

156. Prokop M, Galanski M. *Spiral and Multislice Computed Tomography of the Body.* Stuttgart, Germany: Thieme; 2003.

157. Reimann AJ, Rinck D, Birinci-Aydogan A, et al. Dual-source computed tomography: advances of improved temporal resolution in coronary plaque imaging. *Invest Radiol.* 2007; 42: 196–203.

158. Royal HD. Effects of low level radiation—what's new? *Semin Nucl Med.* 2008; 38:392–402.

159. Shechter G, Koehler Th, Altman A, and Proksa R. The frequency split method for helical cone-beam reconstruction. *Med Phys.* 2004; 31: 2230–2236.

160. Schoder H, Erdi YE, Larson SM, and Yeung HW. PET/CT: a new imaging technology in nuclear medicine. *Eur J Nucl Med Mol Imaging.* 2003; 30:1419–1437.

161. Schueler BA. Incorporating radiation dose assessments into the ACR appropriateness criteria. *J Am Coll Radiol.* 2008; 5:775–776.

162. Schoenhagen P, Stillman AE, Halliburton SS, et al. Non-invasive coronary angiography with multi-detector computed tomography: comparison to conventional X-ray angiography. *Int J Cardiovasc Imaging.* 2005; 21:63–72.

163. Schoepf UJ, Becker CR, Obuchowski NA, et al. Multi-slice computed tomography as a screening tool for colon cancer, lung cancer and coronary artery disease. *Eur Radiol.* 2001; 11: 1975–1985.

164. Schroeder T, Malago M, Debatin JF, et al. "All-in-one" imaging protocols for the evaluation of potential living liver donors: comparison of magnetic resonance imaging and multidetector computed tomography. *Liver Transpl.* 2005; 11:776–787.

165. Seeram E. *Computed Tomography: Physical Principles, Clinical Applications, and Quality Control.* Philadelphia: W.B. Saunders; 2009.

166. Segars WP, Mahesh M, Beck TJ, et al. Realistic CT simulation using the 4D XCAT phantom. *Med Phys.* 2008; 35:3800–3808.

167. Shepp LA, Kruskal JB. Computerized tomography: the new medical x-ray technology. *Am Math Mo.* 1978; 85:420.

168. Shepp LA, Logan EC. The Fourier reconstruction of a head section. *IEEE Trans Nucl Sci.* 1974; 21:2.

169. Shope TB, Gagne RM, Johnson GC. A method for describing the doses delivered by transmission x-ray computed tomography. *Med Phys.* 1981; 8:488–495.

170. Silverman PM, Kalender WA, Hazle JD. Common terminology for single and multislice helical CT. *AJR Am J Roentgenol.* 2001; 176:1135–1136.

171. Smith RA, Cokkinides V, and Brawley OW. Cancer screening in the United States, 2009: a review of current American Cancer Society guidelines and issues in cancer screening. *CA Cancer J Clin.* 2009; 59:27–41.

172. Stierstorfer K, Wolf H, Kuehn U, et al. Principle and Performance of a Dynamic Collimation Technique for Spiral CT. *RSNA Scientific Assembly and Annual Meeting Program* 2007;268.

173. Tack D, De Maertelaer V, Gevenois PA. Dose reduction in multidetector CT using attenuation-based online tube current modulation. *AJR Am J Roentgenol.* 2003; 181:331–334.

174. Taguchi K, Anno H. High temporal resolution for multislice helical computed tomography. *Med Phys.* 2000; 27:861–872.

175. Taguchi K, Aradate H. Algorithm for image reconstruction in multi-slice helical CT. *Med Phys.* 1998; 25:550–561.

176. Taguchi K, Aradate H, Saito Y, Zmora I, Han KS, Silver MD. The cause of the artifact in 4-slice helical computed tomography. *Med Phys.* 2004; 31:2033–2037.

177. Taguchi K, Chiang BS, Hein IA. Direct cone-beam cardiac reconstruction algorithm with cardiac banding artifact correction. *Med Phys.* 2006; 33:521–539.

178. Thibault JB, Sauer KD, Bouman CA, et al. A three-dimensional statistical approach to improved image quality for multislice helical CT. *Med Phys.* 2007; 34:4526–4544.

179. Toth TL, Bromberg NB, Pan TS, et al. A dose reduction x-ray beam positioning system for high-speed multislice CT scanners. *Med Phys.* 2000; 27:2659–2668.

180. Townsend DW. Physical principles and technology of clinical PET imaging. *Ann Acad Med Singapore.* 2004; 33:133–145.

181. Townsend DW, Beyer T. A combined PET/CT scanner: the path to true image fusion. *Br J Radiol.* 2002; 75 Spec No:S24–30.

182. Townsend DW, Beyer T, Blodgett TM. PET/CT scanners: a hardware approach to image fusion. *Semin Nucl Med.* 2003; 33:193–204.

183. Townsend DW, Carney JP, Yap JT, et al. PET/CT today and tomorrow. *J Nucl Med.* 2004; 45(suppl 1):4S–14S.

184. Ulzheimer S, Kalender WA. Assessment of calcium scoring performance in cardiac computed tomography. *Eur Radiol.* 2003; 13:484–497.

185. van der Moolen A and Geleijns J. Overranging in multisection CT: quantification and relative contribution to dose-comparison of four 16-section CT scanners. *Radiol.* 2007; 242:208–216.

186. Wagner LK and Mulhern OR. Radiation-attenuating surgical gloves: effects of scatter and secondary electron production. *Radiol.* 1996; 200:45–48.

187. Wahl RL. Why nearly all PET of abdominal and pelvic cancers will be performed as PET/CT. *J Nucl Med.* 2004; 45(suppl 1):82S–95S.

188. Wessling J, Esseling R, Raupach R, et al. The effect of dose reduction and feasibility of edge-preserving noise reduction on the detection of liver lesions using MSCT. *Eur Radiol.* 2007;17:1885–1891.

189. Weinreb JCL, Woodard PA, Stanford PK, et al. American College of Radiology Clinical Statement on Noninvasive Cardiac Imaging. *Radiology.* 2005; 235:723–727.

190. Wintermark M, Maeder P, Verdun FR, et al. Using 80 kVp versus 120 kVp in perfusion CT measurement of regional cerebral blood flow. *AJNR Am J Neuroradiol.* 2000; 21:1881–1884.

191. Wintersperger BJ, Nikolaou K, von Ziegler F, et al. Image quality, motion artifacts, and reconstruction timing of 64-slice coronary computed tomography angiography with 0.33-second rotation speed. *Invest Radiol.* 2006; 41:436–442.

192. Wrixon AD. New ICRP recommendations. *J Radiol Prot.* 2008; 28:161–168.

193. Wrixon AD. New recommendations from the International Commission on Radiological Protection—a review. *Phys Med Biol.* 2008; 53:R41–60.

194. Nakayama Y, Awai K, Funama Y, et al. Abdominal CT with low tube voltage: preliminary observations about radiation dose, contrast enhancement, image quality, and noise. *Radiology.* 2005; 237:945–951.

195. Yoshizumi TT, Goodman PC, Frush DP, et al. Validation of metal oxide semiconductor field effect transistor technology for organ dose assessment during CT: comparison with thermoluminescent dosimetry. *AJR Am J Roentgenol.* 2007; 188:1332–1336.

196. Zatz L, ed. *General Overview of Computed Tomography Instrumentation.* St. Louis: Mosby; 1981.

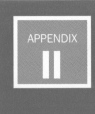

APPENDIX

II

Table A.1 Radiation quantities and units

Quantity	Conventional unit	SI unit	Conversions
Exposure[a]	Roentgen (R)	C/Kg	1 C/Kg = 3876 R (1 R = 2.58 × 10 C/Kg)
Absorbed dose[b]	rad	Gray (Gy)	1 Gy = 100 rad
Effective dose[c]	rem	Sievert (Sv)	1 Sv = 100 rem

[a] Amount of charge created by ionizing radiation per unit volume in air.
[b] Energy deposited per unit mass of material by radiation.
[c] Permits comparisons of radiation with differing biological effects.

Table A.2 Conversion tables for effective dose and organ dose values between Standard International (SI) units and conventional units

Effective doses	Organ doses
1 Sv = 100 rem	1 Gy = 100 rad
100 mSv = 10 rem	100 mGy = 10 rad
10 mSv = 1 rem	10 mGy = 1 rad
1 mSv = 0.1 rem = 100 mrem	1 mGy = 0.1 rad = 100 mrad
0.1 mSv = 0.01 rem = 10 mrem	0.1 mGy = 0.01 rad = 10 mrad
0.01 mSv = 0.001 rem = 1 mrem	0.02 mGy = 0.001 rad = 1 mrad
0.001 mSv = 1 μSv = 0.1 mrem	0.001 mGy = 1 μGy = 0.1 mrad

[a] 0.01–50 mSv (1 mrem to 5 rem) = typical range of effective doses observed in medical x-ray imaging protocols, including MDCT protocols.

Table A.3 Organ or tissue weighting factors (w_T) for estimating effective dose in CT

Organ or tissue	Weighting factor	
	ICRP 60	ICRP 103[a]
Breast	**0.05**	**0.12**
Red bone marrow, colon, lung, stomach	0.12	0.12
Remainder tissues[b]	0.05	0.12
Gonads	**0.20**	**0.08**
Bladder, liver, thyroid, esophagus	0.05	0.04
Skin, bone surface	0.01	0.01
Brain and salivary glands		0.01

Effective dose values estimated for CT protocols are currently based on organ or tissue weighting factors from ICRP publication 60 (International Council of Radiation Protection) published in 1991. ICRP 103 (published in 2007) has certain organ or tissue weighting factors modified. This will have impact on the effective dose estimations, especially for CT protocols in the chest and pelvis regions.
[a] Wrixon AD. New ICRP recommendations. *J Radiol Protect* 2008;28:161–168.
[b] Accounts additional tissues/organs such as adernals, kidney, small and large intestine, muscle, pancreas, spleen, thymus, and uterus.

Table A.4 Adult effective doses for various CT procedures[*]

Examination	Effective dose (mSv)	Range in literature (mSv)
Head	2	0.9 – 4.0
Neck	3	…
Chest	7	4.0–18.0
Chest for pulmonary embolism	15	13–40
Abdomen	8	3.5–25
Pelvis	6	3.3–10
Three-phase liver study	15	…
Spine	6	1.5–10
Coronary angiography	16	5.0–32
Calcium scoring	3	1.0–12
Virtual colonoscopy	10	4.0–13.2

[*] Mettler FA Jr., Huda W, Yoshizumi TT, Mahesh M. Effective doses in radiology and diagnostic nuclear medicine: a catalog. Radiology 2008;248:254–263.

Index

Page numbers followed by *f* and *t* indicate figures and tables